CANCER PAIN

CURRENT MANAGEMENT OF PAIN

P. PRITHVI RAJ, SERIES EDITOR

The series, *Current Management of Pain*, is intended by the series editor and the publishers to provide up-to-date information on advances in the clinical management of acute and chronic pain and related research as quickly as possible. Both the series editor and the publishers felt that, although comprehensive texts are now available, they do not always cover the rapid advances in this field. Another format was needed to publish advances in basic sciences and clinical modalities and to bring them rapidly to the practitioners in the community. A questionnaire was sent to selected clinicians and, based on their responses, topics were chosen by the series editor. Editors of each volume were chosen for their expertise in the field and their ability to encourage other active pain specialists to contribute their knowledge.

Ghia JN (ed): The Multidisciplinary Pain Center: Organization and Personnel Functions for Pain Management 1988. ISBN 0-89838-359-5.

Lynch TN, Vasudevan SV (eds): Persistent Pain: Psychosocial Assessment and Intervention. 1988. ISBN 0-89838-363-3.

Abram SE (ed): Cancer Pain, 1988. ISBN 0-89838-389-7.

CANCER PAIN

Distributors for North America:
Kluwer Academic Publishers
101 Philip Drive
Assinippi Park
Norwell, Massachusetts 02061 USA

Distributors for the UK and Ireland:
Kluwer Academic Publishers
Falcon House, Queen Square
Lancaster LA1 1RN, UNITED KINGDOM

Distributors for all other countries:
Kluwer Academic Publishers
Distribution Centre
Post Office Box 322
3300 AH Dordrecht, THE NETHERLANDS

Library of Congress Cataloging-in-Publication Data
Cancer pain/edited by Stephen E. Abram.
        p.   cm.—(Current management of pain; 3)
    Includes index.
    ISBN-13:978-1-4612-8223-5   e-ISBN-13:978-1-4613-0875-1
    DOI:10.1007/978-1-4613-0875-1

    1. Cancer pain—Treatment.   2. Analgesia.   I. Abram, Stephen E.   II. Series.
    [DNLM: 1. Neoplasms—physiopathology.   2. Neoplasms—therapy.   3. Pain—therapy.
QZ 266 C2162]
RC262.C291182 1988
616.99′4—dc19
DNLM/DLC
for Library of Congress   88-12926
                                                                                CIP

CONTENTS

Pain due to cancer has always provoked despair and depression in patients while, in physicians, empathy and a strong dedication to improving the quality of life in such dying patients. One would think that the goal of pain relief was achievable, since tremendous advances have been made in the last quarter of a century in developing new and powerful analgesics, improved techniques of administration, hospice programs, and home care. This unfortunately is not everywhere the case.

Of the 5 million patients who suffer from cancer globally approximately, 58% complain of intolerable pain in a random survey. As they approach the terminal stage, this increases to 85%. The knowledge that they have cancer produces havoc in their physical and emotional life. Initially, there is denial, followed by anger, depression, and fear. Their physical and mental strength deteriorates rapidly and they withdraw from society into their own world of suffering. To take them out of this world of suffering, one has to deal not only with relief of nociception but also to alter the psychological and biosocial changes that almost certainly occur. A monograph on cancer pain management, then, should obviously include updated techniques in alleviating not only nociception but also psychobiosocial changes.

The series editor and the publishers have been fortunate, indeed, to have Dr. Stephen Abrams accept this task. He has impeccable credentials. He is in the forefront of pain medicine in the United States today, actively participating in care of pain patients as well as developing standards of pain treatments. He has devoted his entire professional life to caring for cancer patients. His mission has been to provide the latest advances in pain relief techniques for cancer patients. He has selected authors of international repute to accomplish this. A look at the contents will suffice to note that he has achieved this task admirably. It is the hope of the series editor and the publisher that the reader will find this monograph informative, current, and enlightening.

P. Prithvi Raj

Dedication

This book is dedicated to all people whose final experiences with life have been needlessly distorted by cancer pain. It is dedicated as well to Ernest O. Henschel, M.D., who faced his last days as he faced his life: with courage and dignity.

CONTRIBUTING AUTHORS

Stephen E. Abram, M.D.
Professor and Vice Chairman, Department of Anesthesiology
Medical College of Wisconsin
Director, Pain Clinic
Milwaukee County Medical Complex
8700 West Wisconsin Avenue
Milwaukee, WI 53226

Ross A. Abrams, M.D.
Assistant Professor, Department of Radiation Oncology
Medical College of Wisconsin
8700 West Wisconsin Avenue
Milwaukee, WI 53226

Sheldon L. Burchman, M.D.
Associate Clinical Professor, Department of Anesthesiology
Director, St. Mary's Hospice
Medical College of Wisconsin
8700 West Wisconsin Avenue
Milwaukee, WI 53226

Charles S. Cleeland, Ph.D.

Professor, Department of Neurology
Director, Pain Research Group
University of Wisconsin School of Medicine
600 Highland Avenue, H6/530
Madison, WI 53792

Dennis W. Coombs, M.D.
Associate Professor, Section of Anesthesiology
Director, Pain Management Service
Dartmouth–Hitchcock Medical Center
Hanover, NH 03755

Theresa Ferrer-Brechner, M.D.
Professor, Department of Anesthesiology
Director, Pain Management Center
UCLA Medical Center
10833 Leconte Avenue
Los Angeles, CA 90024

Richard M. Hansen, M.D.
Associate Professor, Department of Medicine
Section of Hematology–Oncology
Medical College of Wisconsin
8700 West Wisconsin Avenue
Milwaukee, WI 53226

Sanford J. Larson, M.D., Ph.D.
Professor and Chairman, Department of Neurosurgery
Medical College of Wisconsin
8700 West Wisconsin Avenue
Milwaukee, WI 53226

Richard Payne, M.D.
Associate Professor, Department of Neurology
University of Cincinnati Medical Center
231 Bethesda
Cincinnati, OH 45267-0525

Charles W. Quimby, Jr., M.D., LL.B.
Associate Professor, Department of Anesthesiology
Vanderbilt University Medical School
Nashville, TN 37232

Patrick R. Walsh, M.D.
Associate Professor, Department of Neurosurgery
Medical College of Wisconsin
8700 West Wisconsin Avenue
Milwaukee, WI 53226

PREFACE

The diagnosis of cancer inspires fear, in part because of the high mortality rate associated with most malignancies, and in part because of the perception that cancer is a painful disease. Recently compiled statistics tend to support patients' fears. Pain is a major symptom in 70% of patients with advanced cancer [1]. Half of all patients undergoing anticancer therapy experience pain [2]. It has been estimated by members of the World Health Organization that 3.5 million people worldwide suffer from cancer pain. One study of the severity of cancer pain estimates that pain is moderate to severe in 50% of cancer pain patients, very severe or excruciating in 30% [3]. An analysis of several reports of patients in developed countries estimates that 50–80% of patients had inadequate relief [2]. In underdeveloped countries, adequacy of treatment may be far lower because of lack of availability of medical facilities and legal constraints on the use of potent narcotics.

The picture need not be this bleak. The reality is that, for most patients, cancer pain is relatively easy to control with simple, inexpensive measures. Several studies have indicated that cancer pain can be well controlled with oral morphine in over 90% of patients [4,5]. Long-acting orally effective opiate preparations such as time-release morphine, methadone, and levorphanol allow patients to sleep comfortably through the night. When the oral route is impossible, narcotics can be administered rectally or by intravenous or subcutaneous infusion. Patient-controlled analgesia eliminates delays in delivery of prn medications. Some newer preparations can be given transdermally or sublingually. When systemic opiates are ineffective, the epidural, subarachnoid, or intracerebroventricular routes may be dramatically effective. A variety of nonopiate medications may greatly enhance the efficacy of narcotics. Radiation therapy, chemotherapy, and hormonal therapy provide profound relief of pain for certain types of malignancy. For particularly troublesome cases we can turn to neurolytic blockade, cryoanalgesic procedures, ablative neurosurgery, or neurostimulation procedures.

With the majority of cancer pain patients responsive to simple analgesic measures, and with the availability of an impressive array of techniques for resistant cases, why do so many cancer patients suffer severe pain? Inadequate treatment by health care professionals is the primary reason. A study by Marks and Sachar [6] showed that many physicians underprescribed analgesic medications. In addition, most patients received only 20–25% of the amount prescribed. Fear that patients will become addicted or will stop breathing are common barriers to the administration of adequate doses. A nurse may give only a portion of a prescribed narcotic order if she feels the dose is excessive. When a range of doses is ordered, the low end of the range is almost invariably administered. Inadequate knowledge of the pharmacology of analgesic agents is widespread among physicians and nurses. Drugs with a two- to three-hour duration are commonly administered at four- to six-hour intervals. When tolerance develops to the analgesic effect of opiates, health care providers may not understand that patients also become tolerant to the side effects and are often reluctant to escalate doses to appropriate levels.

Increasing regulatory requirements and physician surveillance regarding prescribing of scheduled drugs tends to discourage adequate utilization. Pharmacies may be undersupplied with opiate drugs because of infrequent use or fears of theft and violence. Patient compliance may be poor because of fears of addiction, or concern that taking strong drugs too early will limit efficacy later in the disease. In many countries, potent oral narcotic preparations are simply not available to the medical community.

Undertreatment of pain is not the only disservice we provide for cancer patients. Aggressive treatment with neurodestructive nerve blocks and surgical procedures is often carried out without adequate trials of less risky procedures. Dr. Sheldon Burchman's frequently voiced warning is appropriate to this situation: "Your patient will not thank you for destroying his bladder and bowel control and depriving him of his last shred of human dignity." We must attempt to relieve pain with the least risk to the patient and the least interference with his remaining life.

Adequate management of cancer pain can be accomplished only if the following requirements are met by health care providers:

1. Recognition of the patient's pain. Nurses and physicians must actively question their patients about their pain, and must accept the patient's assessment of its severity and adequacy of control.
2. Understanding of the source and mechanisms of the pain.
3. Knowledge of the pharmacology of analgesics and adjuvants.
4. Willingness to use adequate analgesic doses and to adjust doses frequently.

5. Knowledge of the entire spectrum of treatment options available for resistant problems.
6. Use of an organized management scheme, with progression from low-risk, low-discomfort strategies to high-risk, more invasive treatments as required.

A multidisciplinary approach to cancer pain management is helpful for resistant and complicated problems. While such an approach has come into vogue in the treatment of chronic noncancer pain, few centers have adapted the multidisciplinary approach to cancer pain management, despite the difficulty and complexity of the problems encountered. The oncologist, radiation therapist, anesthesiologist, neurosurgeon, psychiatrist or psychologist, and oncology nurse should be regular members of such a team. Management schemes should concentrate on providing patients with maximum comfort while minimizing procedural risk, cost, and discomfort. Staffing conferences on difficult patients allows the management team to judge the potential risk and efficacy of various treatment options for a particular patient.

It is the purpose of this volume to explore the range of cancer pain management techniques available to health care professionals and their patients. An understanding of the potential benefits and the possible risks and discomfort of pain treatment options is essential for all physicians and nurses who care for patients with malignant disease. It is the sincere wish of the editor and the chapter authors that publication of this material will promote an increase in interest, awareness, and expertise in cancer pain management that will lead to a reduction in unnecessary patient suffering.

Stephen E. Abram, M.D.

REFERENCES

1. Bonica JJ (1985): Treatment of cancer pain: current status and future needs. In: Fields HL et al. (eds), Advances in Pain Research and Therapy, vol 9. New York: Raven Press, pp 589–616.
2. Foley KM (1979): The management of pain of malignant origin. In: Tyler HR, Dawson DM (eds), Current Neurology, vol 2. Boston: Houghton Mifflin, pp 279–302.
3 Daut RT, Cleeland CS (1982): The prevalence and severity of pain in cancer. Cancer 50:1913–1918.
4. Melzack R, Ofiesh JG, Mount BM (1976): The Brompton Mixture: effects on pain in cancer patients. Canad Med Ass J 115:122–126.
5. Saunders CM (1978): The management of terminal disease. In: Saunders CM (ed), Management of Malignant Disease. London: Edward Arnold, p 16.
6. Marks RM, Sachar EJ (1973): Undertreatment of medical inpatients with narcotic analgesics. Ann Int Med 78:173–181.

1. CANCER PAIN MECHANISMS AND ETIOLOGY

RICHARD PAYNE, M.D.

MAJOR CATEGORIES OF PAIN IN CANCER

Pain associated with cancer may result from tumor infiltration of pain-sensitive structures, injury to nerves, bone, and soft tissue as a result of chemotherapy, radiotherapy, or surgery, and tumor or radiation-induced vascular occlusion (table 1-1) [8,15]. One can distinguish three basic categories or types of pain: somatic, visceral and deafferentation (table 1-2).

Somatic or nociceptive pain occurs as a result of tissue injury with resultant activation of nociceptors in cutaneous and deep tissues. This pain is typically well localized and is generally well managed by cancer treatment (e.g., radiation therapy) and analgesic drugs. Examples of somatic pain include bone metastasis [14], postsurgical incisional pain, and myofascial or musculoskeletal pain.

Visceral pain is also common in the cancer patient, and results from infiltration, compression, distention, or stretching of thoracic and abdominal viscera, usually as a result of primary or metastatic tumor growth (e.g., liver metastasis and pancreatic cancer). This type of pain is poorly localized, often described as "deep," "squeezing," and "pressure," and may be associated with nausea, vomiting, and diaphoresis, particularly when acute. Visceral pain is often referred to cutaneous sites that may be remote from the site of the lesion (e.g., shoulder pain with diaphragmatic irritation), and may be associated with tenderness in the referred cutaneous site.

Deafferentation pain, the third major type of pain, results from injury to the peripheral and/or central nervous systems as a consequence of tumor compression or

Table 1-1. Specific pain syndromes in patients with cancer

Pain Syndromes Associated with Direct Tumor Infiltration
Tumor infiltration of bone
  Base of skull syndromes
    Jugular foramen metastases
    Clivus metastases
    Sphenoid sinus metastases
  Vertebral body syndromes
    C2 metastases
    C7, T1 metastases
    L1 metastases
  Sacral syndrome
Tumor infiltration of nerve
  Peripheral nerve
    Peripheral neuropathy
  Plexus
    Brachial plexopathy
    Lumbar plexopathy
    Sacral plexopathy
  Root
    Leptomeningeal metastases
  Spinal cord
    Epidural spinal cord compression
Pain Syndromes Associated with Cancer Therapy
Postsurgery syndromes
  Postthoracotomy syndrome
  Postmastectomy syndrome
  Postradical neck syndrome
  Phantom limb syndrome
Postchemotherapy syndromes
  Mucositis and pharyngitis[a]
  Peripheral neuropathy
  Aseptic necrosis of the femoral head
  Steroid pseudorheumatism
  Postherpetic neuralgia
Postradiation syndromes
  Pharyngitis and esophagitis[a]
  Radiation fibrosis of brachial and lumbar plexus
  Radiation myelopathy
  Radiation-induced second primary tumors
  Radiation necrosis of bone
Pain Syndromes Not Associated with Cancer of Cancer Therapy
Osteoporosis
Cervical and lumbar osteoarthritis
Thoracic and abdominal aneurysms
Diabetic neuropathy

---

[a] Usually self-limited.
Adapted from: Payne R, Foley KM (1984): Recent advances in cancer pain management. Cancer Treatment Reports 68:173–183.

Table 1-2. Types of cancer-related pain

	Somatic	Visceral	Deafferentation
Characteristics of pain	Constant; aching; gnawing; well localized	Constant; aching; poorly localized; often referred to cutaneous sites	Paroxysms of pain "shooting or shock-like" on background of burning, aching sensations
Putative mechanisms	Activation of nociceptors	Activation of nociceptors	Spontaneous and paroxysmal discharges in the PNS and CNS
Examples	Bone metastasis	Pancreatic cancer Liver/lung mets with shoulder pain	Metastatic brachial and lumbosacral plexopathies
Management of pain	Treat tumor Analgesics TENS[a] Nerve blocks Cordotomy	Treat tumor Analgesics Nerve blocks ?Cordotomy	Analgesics (esp. adjuvants) TENS[a] ?Nerve blocks (including sympathetic blocks) ?Treat tumor

[a] TENS = transcutaneous electrical nerve stimulation.

infiltration of peripheral nerve or the spinal cord, or trauma or chemical injury to peripheral nerve as a result to surgery, radiation, or chemotherapy for cancer [15,56,63]. Examples of deafferentation pain include metastatic or radiation-induced brachial or lumbosacral plexopathies, epidural spinal cord and/or cauda equina compression, post herpetic neuralgia, and painful vincristine or cis-platinum neuropathy [15,24,25,56]. Pain resulting from neural injury is often severe, and is different in quality as compared to somatic or visceral pain [56]. It is typically described as a constant dull ache, often with a pressure or "viselike" quality; superimposed paroxysms of burning and/or electrical shocklike sensations are common [3,56]. These paroxysms of pain may be associated with spontaneous and ectopic activity in the peripheral and central nervous systems occurring as a consequence of nerve injury [3,10,11,55].

The sympathetic nervous system may be involved in these pain states (particularly acute visceral and deafferentation pain), although its role is poorly understood [39,41]. Evidence for the involvement of the sympathetic nervous system in pain include 1) the improvement of some forms of pain with sympathetic nerve blocks [33] or with adrenergic blocking drugs such as propranolol and phenoxybenzamine [18,44]; 2) increase in pain with sympathetic stimulation in some patients with causalgia and other reflex sympathetic dystrophies [61]; and 3) animal studies of peripheral nerve injury that show the development of new alpha-adrenergic receptors and the sensitivity of regenerating nerve sprouts to systemically or locally applied cathecholamines [11].

The following section will describe recent advances in the understanding of the peripheral and central nervous system anatomy, physiology, and pharmacology of nociception. These advances have had direct clinical implications which will be illustrated.

ANATOMY AND PHYSIOLOGY OF CANCER-RELATED PAIN

Nociceptors

Sensory receptors that are preferentially sensitive to noxious (tissue-damaging) or potentially noxious stimuli are prevalent in skin, muscle connective tissues, and thoracic and abdominal viscera [43,65]. These *nociceptors* have been best studied in skin, but many of the physiological properties of cutaneous nociceptors probably apply to visceral and muscle nociceptive units as well [65]. Activation of these units by tumor infiltration of bone and soft tissue is presumed to be a major cause of pain in cancer.

Cutaneous nociceptors

There are several types of cutaneous sensory units in hairy and glaborous (smooth) skin, subcutaneous tissues, and viscera [43]. These units are defined morphologically by their appearance in light and electron microscopy, and physiologically by their patterns of response to mechanical, thermal, and chemical cutaneous stimuli. Once activated, nociceptors conduct impulses via lightly myelinated afferent fibers (A-delta) or unmyelinated (C) afferent fibers [65]. In cutaneous nerves in man, 10% of all myelinated fibers carry nociceptive information; more than 90% of all unmyelinated fibers are nociceptive [20].

The recent discovery and refinement of the technique of microneurography [20,21,57,58,59,60,62] has allowed the stimulation and recording from single afferent or efferent fibers in peripheral nerves of conscious patients or volunteers, and has allowed the correlation of electrical activity in afferent nociceptive fibers with verbal reports of pain [57,59,60]. This is accomplished by inserting tungsten wire with a 2–20μ diameter tip into a single afferent fiber [62]. Microneurographic studies have indicated that activation of a single myelinated nociceptor is sufficient to cause pain, and is associated with sharp, stinging pain [21,58,59,60,62]. Stimulation of unmyelinated nociceptors to discharge frequencies greater than 1.5/second is associated with a dull, burning, or aching pain [57,60].

Other physiological studies in animals and man have demonstrated that nociceptors are not spontaneously active, but may show sensitization, particularly after thermal injury to the skin [20,36]. Sensitization is manifested as 1) a decreased threshold of activation after injury; 2) increased intensity of a response to a noxious injury; and 3) the emergence of spontaneous activity [36]. Sensitization of nociceptors may occur within minutes after a thermal injury, and may last for hours [36]. It has been speculated that this may be the physiological correlate of hyperpathia, which occurs after thermal injury to skin [26], and may be a mechanism of persistent pain in man after various types of tissue damage. Efferent sympathetic activity may also sensitize myelinated nociceptors, although this is unlikely to be a major mechanism of sympathetic involvement in pain [47].

Noncutaneous nociceptors

Pain originating from skeletal muscle, bone, thoracic, abdominal, and pelvic viscera is much more common than cutaneous pain. In the cancer patient, metastatic tumor infiltration of bone, lung, and abdominal viscera is a common cause of pain [7,8,15]. Although much less well studied than their cutaneous counterparts, muscle and visceral nociceptors do exist in almost all organs studied thus far, and appear to have anatomic and physiologic properties similar to cutaneous nociceptors [65].

Tumor metastasis to bone is associated with bone destruction and new bone formation. Myelinated and unmyelinated afferent fibers exist in bone and are in highest density in the periosteum. The bone marrow and cortex of bone are not pain-sensitive, however [7,14]. Prostaglandin synthesis is associated with osteolytic and osteoclastic bone changes in metastasis [17]. Furthermore, prostaglandins E_1 and E_2 (PGE_1/PGE_2) are known to sensitize nociceptors and produce hyperalgesia [13]. Thus, prostaglandin synthesis is thought to be important in the mechanisms of tumor growth and pain in bone metastasis. Corticosteroids and nonsteroidal anti-inflammatory drugs which inhibit prostaglandin synthesis decrease pain and may decrease tumor growth in bone, and therefore have a unique role in management of bone metastasis [9,14,45,53]. Activation of local nociceptors in bone and adjacent peri-articular joints and soft tissue as a result of tumor infiltration may be a common cause of somatic pain in cancer patients.

When normal human viscera are manipulated in conscious patients, pain is usually not elicited, even when the viscera are cut, burned, or crushed [40]. Stimuli that are sufficient to cause visceral pain include 1) irritation of the mucosal and serosal surfaces (e.g., radiation and chemotherapy); 2) torsion or traction of the mesentery; 3) distention or contraction of a hollow viscus (e.g., tumor growth with intralaminal obstruction); and 4) impaction (e.g., dehydration and constipation complicating chemotherapy and narcotic analgesic administration) [29]. Similar stimuli are necessary to provoke pain in the bladder, ureter, or urethra [28,35]. Gastrointestinal nociceptors respond most vigorously to overdistention or contraction of the bowel, and/or torsion of the mesentary—stimuli that are known to cause pain. Afferent fibers from these nociceptors are contained within splanchnic nerves [40].

Visceral pain is often referred to a cutaneous point (which may be tender). Common examples of referred pain in cancer patients include back pain and paraspinal muscle tenderness that occurs with pancreatic and endometrial cancer, right shoulder pain that occurs with hepatoma or liver metastasis, and abdominal or leg pain occurring in prostatic cancer. The mechanism of referred pain is not fully understood, but may be related to convergence of cutaneous and visceral sensory input onto common spinothalamic tract cells in the spinal cord [22,37,48]. It is hypothesized that pain is referred to cutaneous sites because the brain misinterprets the source of sensory input [65]. Another explanation for referred pain is that some afferent fibers innervate both somatic and visceral structures [49]. Thus, activation of visceral nociceptors would cause antidromic activation of cutaneous sensory fibers and could release algesic substances to excite cutaneous nociceptors. There is evidence for both of these mechanisms of referred pain [65].

Summary of neural activity related to cancer pain

Tumor infiltration with associated inflammation and release of algesic chemical mediators in skin, bone, and viscera activate and sensitize nociceptors. This may promote spontaneous and continuous nociceptor activity resulting in persistent pain. Once activated, nociceptors generate impulses that are conducted into the central nervous system via A-delta afferent fibers (thinly myelinated mechanonociceptors) or more slowly conducting C-afferent fibers (unmyelinated polymodal nociceptors responsive to mechanical, thermal, or chemical stimuli). These afferent fibers enter the spinal cord laterally in the dorsal root and synapse in the superficial dorsal horn to activate ascending nociceptive systems (spinothalamic, spinocervical, and spinoreticular tracts), which project to the thalamus and cortex where the stimulus may reach conscious perception as pain.

Injury to afferent nerve fibers or the spinal cord by chemotherapy, radiation therapy, surgery, or metastatic tumor may activate nociceptive systems and produce pain without stimulating nociceptors [41,56]. Pain that occurs as a result of this deafferentation is often qualitatively different from somatic or visceral pain resulting from activation of a nociceptor in the milieu of a *normal* nervous system. Further, deafferentation may produce ectopic or paroxysmal discharges in the peripheral and central nervous system that, in animals, may be associated with pain behaviors [1,2,10]. Similar mechanisms may be operative in man, since deafferentation pain may respond to drugs such as anticonvulsants [34,54], which suppress paroxysmal discharges in nerve, and are generally not useful in somatic or visceral pain.

OPIOID PHARMACOLOGY

Many neurotransmitter systems may be involved in the modulation of nociception, including opioids. In fact, narcotic analgesics are the mainstay of the medical management of severe cancer pain. The endogenous opioid compounds such as enkephalin, β-endorphin, and dynorphin (among others) are among the most potent inhibitors of nociceptive activity within the CNS. Opioids produce dose-dependent suppression of evoked activity in nociceptive and wide-dynamic-range neurons in the CNS [12]. This appears to be an essential feature of opioid analgesic actions [5,6,12]. Opioids reduce the intensity of pain [19,46], and although they have unequivocal effects on mood [27,50], it is controversial as to whether mood effects are primary or secondary to their analgesic effects [19,46].

Endogenous opioids produce analgesia by interacting with specific binding sites, or receptors which are found in high concentration in cortical, brainstem, and spinal cord sites implicated in nociception [4,51]. Narcotic analgesics mimic the action of endogenous opioids by binding to these receptor sites as well. Opioid receptor binding is stereospecific, dose-dependent, and reversed by the antagonist, naloxone [51]. It is now recognized that there are several classes of opioid receptors, which are defined by the pharmacological responses of opioids [23,30,31] or by biochemical binding studies [42]. Thus, one can identify morphine-selective (mu$_2$ receptors), enkephalin-selective (delta receptors), or receptors that bind morphine and enkephalin with about equal affinity (mu_1) [42]. It has been proposed that dynorphin preferentially binds to a kappa opioid receptor subtype [16].

In the doses commonly used in clinical practice, it is likely that the concentration of morphine and other narcotics in the central nervous system is high enough to allow binding to many types of opiate receptors. However, the recognition of multiple opiate receptors with distinct pharmacologic functions [42,68], and their differential anatomical localization within the neuraxis has major implications in the clinical management of cancer pain with narcotic analgesics [67]. For example, it has now been demonstrated that one can separate morphine analgesia (mediated by the mu_1 opiate receptor) from physical dependence [31] and respiratory depression [32] in the rat by the use of irreversible mu_2-receptor-selective antagonist compounds such as naloxonazine. This offers the possibility that mu_1-selective opioids may provide analgesia without these troublesome and occasionally lethal side effects [42]. In fact, meptazinol, a relative mu_1-selective opioid, may be an example of such a drug [52] and is currently in clinical trials.

In addition, it has been demonstrated that opioids with an action limited to the spinal cord may produce analgesia in animals [66] and man [64]. Thus, the epidural or intrathecal administration of small doses of morphine (1–5 mg) produces analgesia and may limit supraspinal side effects, such as respiratory depression and mental clouding [66]. Spinal opioid receptors have a high affinity for delta and kappa ligands [68], and it has recently been determined that the intrathecal administration of d-ala²-d-leu⁵-enkephalin (an analogue of leucine enkephalin and a delta-receptor ligand) may produce analgesia even in morphine-tolerant animals [68] or cancer patients [38].

CONCLUSIONS

The anatomy, physiology, and pharmacology of nociception and its modification by analgesic drugs have been studied extensively in the past decade. Although the neural mechanisms of nociceptors and the stimuli which activate them are much better understood, it must be emphasized that the perception of pain and the meaning of pain to the individual are complex behavioral phenomena and involve psychological and emotional processes in addition to activation of nociceptive pathways.

Pain related to malignant disease can be classified as somatic, visceral, and deafferentation in type. Somatic pain and visceral pain involve direct activation of nociceptors, and are often complications of tumor infiltration of tissues or injury of tissues as a consequence of cancer therapy. The management of this type of pain is typically accomplished by treating the tumor (with surgery, chemotherapy, and/or radiation therapy), and the appropriate use of nonnarcotic, narcotic, and adjuvant analgesic agents. Neuroablative therapies may be helpful in specific circumstances. For example, cordotomy may be helpful for unilateral pain below the waist in patients with somatic and visceral pain. This procedure may also be helpful for early deafferentation pain (e.g., lumbosacral plexopathy), in which peripheral nerves are compressed but not infiltrated or destroyed by metastatic tumor growth.

Deafferentation pain may be a complication of tumor infiltration of peripheral nerve, or a complication of cancer therapy that injures neural tissue [15]. This type of pain is often poorly tolerated and difficult to control, particularly if not treated early and aggressively. Although incompletely understood, the pathophysiology of deafferentation pain appears to be different than that of somatic or visceral pain, and the treatment approaches may be different. Management approaches to deafferentation pain usually emphasize treatment of the pain, because injury to the nervous system may be difficult to reverse, even if one can successfully treat the underlying malignancy, and many deafferentation pain syndromes occur as a complication of cancer therapy. The role of narcotic analgesics in the management of deafferentation pain is not clarified, although the published experience suggests that they are less useful than in somatic or visceral pain [56].

ACKNOWLEDGMENTS

The author is a recipient of a Minority Faculty Development Award from The Robert Wood Johnson Foundation. This work was supported in part by a grant from the National Cancer Institute (3 R18 CA 3289-0351). I thank Marilyn Herleth for her assistance in the preparation of this manuscript.

REFERENCES

1. Albe-Fessard D, Lombard MC (1983): Use of an animal model to evaluate the origin of and protection against deafferentation pain. In: Bonica JJ et al. (eds), Advances in Pain Research and Therapy, vol 5. New York: Raven Press, pp 691–700.
2. Albe-Fessard D, Condes-Lara M, Sanderson P, et al. (1984): Tentative explanation of the special role played by the areas of paleospinothalamic projection in patients with deafferentation pain syndromes. In: Kruger L, Liebskind JC (eds), Neural Mechanisms of Pain (Advances in Pain Research and Therapy, vol 6). New York: Raven Press, pp 167–182.
3. Asbury AK, Fields HL (1984): Pain due to peripheral nerve damage: An hypothesis. Neurology 34:1587–1590.
4. Atweh SF, Kuhar MJ (1977): Autoradiographic localization of opiate receptors in the rat brain. I. Spinal Cord and Lower Medulla. Brain Res 124:53–67.
5. Basbaum AI, Fields HF (1978): Endogenous pain control mechanisms: Review and hypothesis. Ann Neurol 4:451–462.
6. Basbaum AI (1983): The generation and control of pain. In: Rosenberg RN (ed), The Clinical Neurosciences, vol 5. New York: Churchill Livingstone, pp 301–324.
7. Bonica JJ (1953): The Management of Pain. Philadelphia: Lea and Febiger, p 48.
8. Bonica JJ (1985): Treatment of cancer pain: Current status and future needs. In: Fields HL, Dubner R, Cervero F (eds), Advances in Pain Research and Therapy, vol 9. New York: Raven Press, pp 589–616.
9. Brodie GN (1974): Indomethacin and bone pain. Lancet i:1160.
10. Culp WJ, Ochoa J (1982): Abnormal Nerves and Muscles as Impulse Generators. New York: Oxford University Press.
11. Devor M (1983): Nerve pathophysiology and mechanisms of pain in causalgia. J Auton Nerv Syst, 7:371–384.
12. Duggan AW, North RA (1983): Electrophysiology of opioids. Pharmacol Rev, 35:219–282.
13. Ferreira SH, Nakamura M, Castro MSA (1978): The hyperalgesic effects of prostacyclin and prostaglandin E_2. Prostaglandins 16:31–37.
14. Foley KM (1981): Analgesic management of bone pain. In: Weiss L, Gilbert HA (eds), Bone Metastasis. Boston: G.K. Hall Medical Publishers, pp 348–368.
15. Foley KM (1985): The treatment of cancer pain. N Engl J Med 313:84–95.
16. Fredrickson RCA (1984): Endogenous opioids and related derivatives. In: Kuhar M, Pasternak G

(eds), Analgesics: Neurochemical, Behavioral and Clinical Perspectives. New York: Raven Press, pp 9–68.

17. Galasko CSB (1976): Mechanism of bone destruction in the development of skeletal metastasis. Nature 263:507–510.

18. Ghostine SY, Comair YG, Turner DM, et al. (1984): Phenoxybenzamine in the treatment of causalgia. J Neurosurg 60:1263–1268.

19. Gracely RH, McGrath P, Dubner T (1979): Narcotic analgesia: Fentanyl reduces the intensity but not the unpleasantness of painful tooth pulp sensations. Science 203:1261–1263.

20. Hagbarth K-E (1979): Exteroceptive, proprioceptive, and sympathetic activity recorded with microelectrodes from human peripheral nerves. Mayo Clin Proc 54:353–365.

21. Hagbarth K-E, Torebjork HE, Wallin BG (1984): Microelectrode recordings from human skin and muscle nerves. In: Dyck PJ, Thomas PK, Lambert EH et al., Peripheral Neuropathy, vol 1, 2nd edition. Philadelphia: W.B. Saunders Co., pp 1016–1029.

22. Head H (1893): On disturbances of sensation with especial reference to pain of visceral disease. Brain 16:1–132.

23. Iwamoto ET, Martin WR (1981): Multiple opiate receptors. Med Res Rev 1:411–440.

24. Jaeckle KA, Young DF, Foley KM (1985): The natural history of lumbosacral plexopathy in cancer. Neurology 35:8–15.

25. Kori SH, Foley KM, Posner JB (1981): Brachial plexus lesions in patients with cancer: 100 cases. Neurology 31:45–50.

26. LaMotte RH, Campbell JN (1978): Comparison of responses of warm and nociceptor afferents in monkey with human judgements of thermal pain. J Neurophysiol 41:509–528.

27. Lasagna L, van Felsinger JM, Beecher HK (1955): Drug-induced mood changes in man. I. Observations on healthy subjects, chronically ill patients and "postaddicts." JAMA 157:1006–1020.

28. Learmouth JR (1931): A contribution to the neurophysiology of the urinary bladder in man. Brain 54:147–176.

29. Leek BF (1972): Abdominal visceral receptors. In: Neil (ed), Handbook of Sensory Physiology, vol 13. Berlin: Springer, pp 113–160.

30. Ling GSF, Pasternak GW (1983): Spinal and supraspinal analgesia in the mouse: The role of opioid binding sites. Brain Res 271:152–156.

31. Ling GSF, Macleod JM, Lee S, et al. (1984): Separation of morphine analgesia from physical dependence. Science 226:462–464.

32. Ling GSF, Spiegel K, Lockhart SH, et al. (1985): Separation of opioid analgesia from respiratory depression: Evidence for different receptor mechanisms. J Pharmacol Exp Ther 232:149–151.

33. Loh L, Nathan PW (1978): Painful peripheral states and sympathetic blocks. J Neurol Neurosurg Psych 41:664–671.

34. Maciewicz R, Bouckoms A, Martin JB (1985): Drug therapy for neuropathic pain. The Clinical Journal of Pain 1:39–49.

35. McLellan AM, Goddell H (1943): Pain from the bladder, ureter, and kidney pelvis. Res Publ Assoc Res Nerv Ment Disease 23:252–262.

36. Meyer RA, Campbell JN (1981): Myelinated nociceptive afferent account for the hyperalgesia that follows a burn to the hand. Science 213:1527–1529.

37. Milne RJ, Foreman RD, Giesler GJ, et al. (1981): Convergence of cutaneous and pelvic visceral nociceptive inputs onto primate spinothalamic neurons. Pain 11:163–181.

38. Moulin DE, Max MB, Kaiko RF, et al. (1985): The analgesic efficacy of intrathecal d-ala^2-d-leu^5-enkephalin in cancer patients with chronic pain. Pain 23:213–221.

39. Nathan PW (1983): Pain and the sympathetic nervous system. J Auton Nerv Syst 7:363–370.

40. Newman PP (1974): Visceral Afferent Functions of the Nervous System. London: Arnold.

41. Ochoa JL, Torebjork E, Marchettini P, et al. (1985): Mechanisms of neuropathic pain: Cumulative observation, new experiments and further speculation. In: Fields HL, Dubner R, Cervero F (eds), Advances in Pain Research and Therapy, vol 9. New York: Raven Press, pp 431–450.

42. Pasternak GW (1986): Multiple mu opiate receptors: Biochemical and pharmacological evidence for multiplicity. Biochem Pharmacol, 35:361–364.

43. Perl ER (1984): Characterization of nociceptors and their activation of neurons in the superficial dorsal horn: First steps for the sensation of pain. In: Kruger L, Liebeskind JC (eds), Neural Mechanisms of Pain (Advances in Pain Research and Therapy, vol 6). New York: Raven Press, pp 23–52.

44. Pleet AB, Tahmans AJ, Jennings JR (1976): Causalgia treatment with propranolol. Neurology 26:375.

45. Powles TJ, Clark SA, Easty DM, et al. (1973): The inhibition by aspirin and indomethacin of osteolytic tumor deposits and hypercalcemia in rats with Walker tumor and its possible application to human breast cancer. Br J Cancer 28:316–321.
46. Price DD, der Gruen AV, Miller J, et al. (1985): A psychophysical analysis of morphine analgesia. Pain 22:261–269.
47. Roberts WJ, Elardo SM (1985): Sympathetic activation of A-delta nociceptors. Somatosens 3:33–44.
48. Ruch TC (1946): Visceral sensation and referred pain. In: Fulton (ed): Howell's Textbook of Physiology, 15th edition. Philadelphia: Saunders, pp 385–401.
49. Sinclair DC, Weddel G, Feindel WH (1948): Referred pain and associated phenomena. Brain 71:184–211.
50. Smith GM, Beecher HK (1962): Objective evidence of mental effects of heroin, morphine and placebo in normal subjects. J Pharmacol Exp Ther 136:53–58.
51. Snyder SH (1977): Opiate receptors in the brain. N Engl J Med, 296:266–271.
52. Spiegel K, Pasternak GW (1984): Meptazinol: A novel mu-1 selective opioid analgesic. J Pharm Exp Ther 228:414–419.
53. Stoll BA (1973): Indomethacin and breast cancer. Lancet i:384.
54. Swerdlow M (1984): Anticonvulsant drugs and chronic pain. Clin Neuropharmacol 7:51–82.
55. Tasker RR, Tsuda T, Hawrylyshyn (1983): Clinical neurophysiological investigation of deafferentation pain. In: Bonica JJ (ed), Advances in Pain Research and Therapy, vol 5. New York: Raven Press, pp 713–738.
56. Tasker RR (1984): Deafferentation. In: Wall PD, Melzack R (eds), Textbook of Pain. New York: Churchill Livingstone, pp 119–132.
57. Torebjork HE (1979): Activity in C nociceptors and sensation. In: Kenshalo DR (ed): Sensory Function of the Skin of Humans. New York: Plenum Press, pp 313–325.
58. Torebjork HE, Hallin RG (1979): Microneurographic studies of peripheral pain mechanisms in man. In: Bonica JJ (ed), Advances in Pain Research and Therapy, vol 3. New York: Raven Press, pp 121–131.
59. Vallbo AB, Hagbarth K-E, Torebjork HE, et al. (1979): Somatosensory, proprioceptive, and sympathetic activity in human peripheral nerves. Physiol Rev 59:919–957.
60. van Hees J, Gybels JM (1972): Pain related to single afferent C-fibers from human skin. Brain Res 48:397–400.
61. Walker AE, Nulson F (1948): Electrical stimulation of the upper thoracic portion of the sympathetic chain in man. Arch Neurol Psych 5:559–560.
62. Wall PD, McMahon SB (1985): Microneuronography and its relation to perceived sensation. A critical review. Pain 21:209–229.
63. Wall PD (1985): Cancer pain: Neurogenic mechanisms. In: Fields HL, Dubner R, Cervero F (eds), Advances in Pain Research and Therapy, vol 9. New York: Raven Press, pp 575–587.
64. Wang JK, Nauss LA, Thomas JE (1979): Pain relief by intrathecally-applied morphine in man. Anesthesiology 50:149–151.
65. Willis WD (1985): The Pain System: The Neural Basis of Nociceptive Transmission in the Mammalian Nervous System. Basel: S. Karger.
66. Yaksh TL (1981): Spinal opiate analgesia: Characteristics and principles of action. Pain 11:293–347.
67. Yaksh TL, Hammond DL (1982): Peripheral and central substrates involved in the rostrad transmission of nociceptive information. Pain 13:1–85.
68. Yaksh TL (1983): In vivo studies on spinal opiate receptor systems mediating antinociception. I. mu and delta receptor profiles in the primate. J Pharmacol Exp Ther 226:303–316.

2. ORAL AND PARENTERAL DRUG THERAPY FOR CANCER PAIN

RICHARD PAYNE, M.D.

INTRODUCTION

Pain in the cancer patient is often a consequence of tumor infiltration or compression of bone, soft tissue, peripheral nerve or spinal cord, or vascular occlusion [4,17]. The most effective management of cancer pain involves treatment of the tumor with surgery, radiation therapy, or chemotherapy, if possible. However, it is often necessary to manage pain with analgesic drugs prior to the introduction of specific antitumor therapy. Moreover, a significant percentage of patients will have chronic pain as a sequela of cancer treatment [42] (see table 1-1, Chapter 1, this volume). Finally, although invasive neurosurgical and anesthetic approaches to cancer pain management are indicated in a minority of patients, with a few exceptions (e.g., celiac ganglion blocks for pancreatic pain) they are not first-line treatments [16]. Therefore, the use of analgesic drugs has become the mainstay of acute and chronic cancer pain management, and narcotic analgesics are the drugs of choice for management of severe pain [4,15,55].

Although the therapy of cancer pain has improved recently, significant limitations in the optimal management of pain remain. In part, these limitations are imposed by misconceptions and ignorance regarding the clinical pharmacology of analgesic drugs, especially narcotics [4,15]. This chapter will outline guidelines for the use of the three major classes of analgesic drugs, emphasizing the use of narcotics in the management of cancer pain.

The three major classes of analgesic drugs are 1) *aspirin and nonsteroidal anti-*

inflammatory drugs (NSAIDs), which act on peripheral nerve endings at the site of injury, and produce analgesia by altering the prostaglandin system; 2) *adjuvant analgesics*, which act centrally to produce analgesia in certain pain states; and 3) *narcotic analgesics (opioids)*, which act by binding to opiate receptors and activating endogenous pain suppression systems in the CNS. The choice of the specific drug approach is based on an assessment of the pain syndrome, the severity of the pain, and an understanding of the clinical pharmacology of specific analgesics.

NONNARCOTIC ANALGESICS

These agents are useful in mild to moderate cancer pain, especially if related to bone metastasis and musculoskeletal inflammation. These drugs include aspirin, fenoprofen, ibuprofen, diflunisal, and naproxen (see table 2-1). In addition to their actions as analgesics, they have antipyretic, antiplatelet, and anti-inflammatory effects [30]. However, there is a ceiling effect to analgesia. For instance, increasing the dose of aspirin beyond 975–1300 mg/day will produce no increase in peak effect but may increase the duration of analgesia.

In addition to the analgesic ceiling effect, these agents differ from morphine like analgesics in that 1) they do not produce tolerance, or physical or psychological dependence, and 2) their presumed mechanism of action is inhibition of the enzyme prostaglandin synthetase (cyclooxygenase), preventing the synthesis of prostaglandins from arachidonic acid [30]. Prostaglandin E_2 (PGE_2) is known to sensitize nociceptors on peripheral nerves to the pain-producing effects of substances such as bradykinin and other chemical mediators of inflammation [31]. Thus, NSAIDs can influence pain at the level of the peripheral nervous system, and may act synergistically with narcotic analgesics, which modulate pain in the central nervous system. They differ from each other in their pharmacokinetics (e.g., plasma half-lives) and duration of analgesia. Ibuprofen and fenoprofen have short half-lives and the same duration of action as aspirin; diflunisal and naproxen have longer half-lives and are longer-acting than aspirin. Prolongation of the bleeding time may occur due to inhibition of platelet cyclooxygenase and reduced formation of thromboxane A_2. Gastric irritation also occurs commonly with this class of drugs.

Acetaminophen is also grouped in this class. It is roughly equipotent to aspirin in its analgesic and antipyretic potency, but has no anti-inflammatory or antiplatelet effects. Side effects include hepatotoxicity at doses greater than 10–15 grams/day. Choline magnesium trisalicylate is also an effective analgesic, lacks antiplatelet effects, and has fewer gastrointestinal side effects than aspirin.

Nonsteroidal anti-inflammatory analgesics (especially indomethacin) may have a unique role in the management of bone pain secondary to tumor metastasis. However, with the exception of acetaminophen and, perhaps, choline magnesium trisalicylate, the use of NSAIDs in oncology is limited because of their antiyretic effects, which may mask infection in a high-risk population (especially children), and because their effects on platelet function may risk hemorrhage in patients with thrombocytopenia and coagulation defects.

Table 2-1. Analgesics commonly used orally for mild to moderate pain

Name	Equianalgesic Dose (mg)[a]	Oral Dose Range (mg)	Duration of Analgesia (hours)	Plasma Half-Life (hours)	Pediatric Dose[b] (mg/kg/dose)	Comments
A. Nonnarcotics						
Aspirin	650	650 QID	4–6	3–5	10	Standard of comparison for nonnarcotics; often used in combination with narcotic-type analgesics; papillary necrosis and interstitial nephritis with chronic use; avoid during pregnancy, in hemostatic disorders and in combination with steroids
Acetaminophen	650	650 QID	4–6	1–4	10	Like aspirin (but no anti-inflammatory or antiplatelet effects)
Ibuprofen (Motrin®)	—	200–400 QID	4–6	2		Higher analgesic potential than aspirin
Fenoprofen (Nalfon®)	—	200–400 QID	4–6	3		Like ibuprofen
Diflunisal (Dolobid®)	—	500–1000 BID	8–12	8–12		Longer duration of action than ibuprofen; higher analgesic potential than aspirin
Naproxen (Naprosyn®)	—	250–500 QID	8–12	14		Like diflunisal
Choline magnesium salicylate (Trilisate®)	—	500–750 BID, TID	8–12	9–17		Anti-inflammatory potency similar to aspirin; few antiplatelet or G.I. effects
B. Narcotics						
Codeine	32–65	32–65 q4h	4–6	3	0.5–1	"Weak" morphine; often used in combination with nonnarcotic analgesics; biotransformed, in part, to morphine; nausea and sedation common with dose escalation

Table 2-1. (continued)

Name	Equianalgesic Dose (mg)[a]	Oral Dose Range (mg)	Duration of Analgesia (hours)	Plasma Half-Life (hours)	Pediatric Dose[b] (mg/kg/dose)	Comments
Oxycodone	5	5–10 q3h	3–5	—	0.08	Short-acting; also formulated in combination with nonnarcotic analgesics (Percodan, Percocet) which limits dose escalation
Meperidine	50	50–100 q3h	3–5	3–4	0.75	Short-acting; biotransformed to normeperidine, a toxic metabolite; normeperidine ($t_{1/2}$ = 12–16 h) accumulates with repetitive dosing causing CNS excitation; not for patients with impaired renal function receiving monoamine oxidase ihibitors
Propoxyphene HCl (Darvon®) Propoxyphene napsylate (Darvon-N®)	65–130	65–130 q4h	4–6	12	—	"Weak" narcotic; often used in combination with nonnarcotic analgesics; long half-life biotransformed to potentially toxic metabolite (norpropoxyphene); propoxyphene and metabolites accumulate with repetitive dosing; overdose complicated by convulsions
Pentazocine (Talwin®)	50	50–100 q4h	4–6	2–3	0.75	In combination with nonnarcotics; in combination with naloxone to discourage parenteral abuse; may cause psychotomimetic effects; mixed agonist–antagonist and therefore, may precipitate withdrawal in narcotic-dependent patients

[a] These doses are recommended starting doses from which the optimal dose for each patient is determined by titration and maximal dose limited by adverse effects. For nonnarcotic analgesics, relative potency was compared to aspirin. For narcotic analgesics, relative potency was compared to 10 mg i.m. morphine.

[b] See Reference 49.

Adapted from Payne R (1987): Pain. In: Wittes RE (ed), *Manual of Oncologic Therapeutics* Philadelphia: J.B. Lippincott Co.

NARCOTIC ANALGESICS (see tables 2-1 and 2-2)

Narcotic analgesics are used to manage moderate to severe cancer-related pain. Ignorance concerning the clinical pharmacology of opioids as well as misconceptions of patients and physicians regarding the phenomena of tolerance, physical dependence, and psychological dependence (addiction) have combined to limit the effectiveness of these agents in the management of cancer pain [10,15,17,34]. When used by physicians with a firm understanding of the clinical pharmacology of narcotic analgesics, and who are aware of their limitations and side effects, adequate pain control with a minimum of adverse effects can be achieved in the majority of patients with pain from metastatic cancer.

Guidelines for narcotic use in cancer pain management

The following guidelines illustrate principles that provide a basis for the rational use of narcotics to manage cancer pain.

Individualize dosage

1. The optimal analgesic dose varies widely among patients. For mild to moderate pain, codeine (30–60 mg p.o. q4h) or oxycodone (Percocet®, 1–2 tablets (5–10 mg of oxycodone) p.o. q4h) are commonly used (see table 2-1). For moderate to severe pain, the typical starting dose for morphine ranges from 5–15 mg (s.c. or i.m.) or 30–60 mg p.o. q3–4h (see table 2-2).

2. Give each analgesic an adequate trial by dose titration (i.e., increasing the dose up to the appearance of limiting side effects) before switching to another drug.

3. Gear the route of administration to the patient's needs, but use the oral route whenever possible. The oral route is convenient and probably associated with a slower rate of tolerance as compared to parenteral routes of administration. However, the onset of pain relief is generally slower after oral administration, and drugs are subject to a *first-pass* effect (i.e., metabolism in the gut wall and liver), thereby reducing their potency. Other routes of administration include sublingual, continuous subcutaneous and intravenous infusion, spinal epidural and intrathecal injections and infusions, and intraventricular. (See section on Novel Routes of Opioid Administration for discussion of indications, dose ranges, and possible complications for each of these routes of administration.)

Administer analgesic regularly (not prn)

Continuous pain requires continuous analgesics. However, this should be done after establishing the optimal dose by titration (especially when using a long half-life drug such as levorphanol or methadone (see table 2-2)). Once the dose requirements for a 24-hour period have been established, the analgesics can be administered on an around-the-clock basis with fewer side effects.

Recognize and treat side effects appropriately

Among the more important side effects are sedation, constipation, nausea, vomiting, and respiratory depression. Narcotic-related sedation is best treated by reducing the

Table 2-2. Narcotic-type analgesics commonly used for severe pain

Name	Equianalgesic I.M. Dose[a] (mg)	I.M./P.O. Potency Ratio	Starting Oral Dose Range (mg)	Pediatric Dose Ranges[b] (mg/kg/dose) I.M.	P.O.	Plasma Half-Life (hours)	Comments
A. Morphinelike agonists							
Morphine	10	6	30–60	0.1–0.2	0.5–1.2	2–3	Standard of comparison for narcotic-type analgesics; lower doses for aged patients with impaired ventilation; bronchial asthma; increased intracranial pressure; liver failure
Hydromorphone (Dilaudid®)	1.5	5	4–8	0.015–0.3	0.04–0.08	2–3	Slightly shorter-acting than morphine; high potency I.M. dosage form for tolerant patients
Methadone (Dolophine®)	10	2	5–20	.0.1–0.2	0.2–0.4	24–36	Good oral potency: long plasma half-life; may accumulate with repetitive dosing causing excessive sedation (on days 2–5)
Levorphanol (Levo-Dromoran®)	2	2	2–4			12–16	Like methadone, may accumulate on days 2–3; delirium and hallucinations may occur
Oxymorphone (Numorphan®)	1	—	—			—	Not available orally; like I.M. morphine
Heroin	5	6–10	—			0.5	Slightly shorter-acting than morphine; biotransformed to active metabolites (e.g., morphine); not available in the U.S.
Meperidine (Demerol®)	75	4	—			3–4	Slightly sorter-acting than morphine; used orally for less severe pain (see table 2-1); toxic metabolite, normeperidine, accumulates with repetitive dosing causing CNS excitation; not for patients with impaired renal function or receiving monoamine oxidase inhibitors

B. Mixed agonist–antagonists				
Pentazocine (Talwin®)	60	3	50–100	2–3	Used orally for less severe pain; ?less abuse liability than morphine; included in Schedule IV of Controlled Substances Act; may cause psychotomimetic effects; may precipitate withdrawal in narcotic-dependent patients; not for myocardial infarction
Nalbuphine (Nubain®)	10	—	—	5	Not available orally; like I.M. pentazocine but not scheduled; incidence of psychotomimetic effects lower with pentazocine
Butorphanol (Stadol®)	2	—	—	2–4	Not available orally; like nalbuphine
C. Partial agonists					
Buprenorphine (Temgesic®)	0.4	—	—	—	Not available orally; sublingual preparation not yet in U.S.; less abuse liability than morphine; does not produce psychotomimetic effects; may precipitate withdrawal in narcotic-dependent patients

For these equianalgesic I.M. doses, the time of peak analgesia in nontolerant patients ranges from one-half to one hour and the duration from four to six hours. The peak analgesic effect is delayed and the duration prolonged after oral administration.

[a] These doses are recommended starting I.M. doses from which the optimal dose for each patient is determined by titration and the maximal dose limited by adverse effects. Equianalgesic doses are based on single-dose studies in which an intramuscular dose of each drug listed was compared with morphine to establish relative potency.

[b] See Reference 49.

Adapted from Payne R (1987): Pain. In: Wittes RE (ed). *Manual of Oncologic Therapeutics* Philadelphia: J.B. Lippincott Co.

dose and increasing the frequency of administration. This avoids high peak concentrations of drug in the brain and may ameliorate sedation, especially when intermittent i.m. or i.v. injections are being used. Dextroamphetamine (5–15 mg/day, p.o.) may be added to increase alertness if the above strategy is unsuccessful and pain is well controlled but the patient is unable to function because of sedation. All patients taking narcotic analgesics will be constipated and should be given stool softeners and laxatives. A useful laxative regimen includes dioctyl sodium sulfosuccinate (Colace®) 100–300 mg/day, and Senokot tablets or suppositories that stimulate colonic motility. Nausea and vomiting may be treated by administering antiemetics (hydroxyzine or a phenothiazine) or by switching to another opiate. Tolerance may develop to the emetic effects of narcotics as well. The appropriate management of respiratory depression will be detailed below.

Use drug combinations that will enhance analgesia

These include narcotics combined with acetaminophen and/or NSAIDs and narcotics combined with miscellaneous adjuvant drugs (see section on adjuvant analgesics).

Distinguish between tolerance, physical dependence, and addiction

Watch for the development of tolerance and treat appropriately. Be aware of the development of physical dependence and prevent withdrawal. Finally, do not confuse the concepts of tolerance, physical dependence, and psychological dependence (or addiction).

Tolerance is an operational term that means that a larger dose of narcotic analgesic is required to maintain the original effect. Tolerance may develop in all patients taking narcotic analgesics for more than one to two weeks. The degree to which tolerance occurs in cancer patients is controversial [14,54]. Tolerance usually occurs in association with physical dependence, but does *not* imply *psychological dependence*. The first sign of the development of tolerance is a decrease in the duration of effective analgesia. However, in patients with cancer, increasing requirements for analgesics are usually also associated with progression of disease. The following strategies may be implemented to delay the development of tolerance and to provide effective analgesia in the tolerant patient: 1) combine narcotics with nonnarcotics; 2) switch to an alternative narcotic and select one-half of the predicted equianalgesic dose given in tables 2-1 and 2-2 as the starting dose, since cross-tolerance among narcotics is not complete; 3) use the oral route in preference to parenteral routes. The above strategies are helpful because tolerance appears to be a function of the dose, frequency, and perhaps route of administration. Thus, intravenous and spinal infusions of narcotics may be associated with rapid dose escalation, suggesting rapid development of tolerance [22,46].

Physical dependence is revealed in patients taking chronic opioids (usually longer than two weeks) when the abrupt discontinuation of a narcotic or the administration of a narcotic antagonist produces an abstinence syndrome. This syndrome is characterized by anxiety, nervousness, irritability, chills alternating with hot flashes, salivation, lacrimation, rhinorrhea, diaphoresis, piloerection, nausea, vomiting, abdominal cramps, insomnia, and, rarely, multifocal myoclonus. The time course of this abstinence syndrome is a function of the half-life of the narcotic. With short half-life drugs such as morphine or hydromorphone, the symptoms may appear in 6–12 hours and peak at 24–72 hours; for methadone and levorphanol (long half-life drugs), the symptoms may be delayed for several days, and are typically less florid. The abstinence syndrome can be avoided by slowly withdrawing chronically used narcotics—about 25% of the previous daily dose is required to prevent withdrawal [16]. This may be necessary when cancer patients receive effective antitumor treatments that relieve the cause of pain, and/or neurosurgical procedures such as cordotomy to control pain so that narcotic analgesic requirements are lowered.

Patients receiving chronic opioids are often tolerant to the respiratory-depressant effects of these agents. In patients who have received a relative overdose of a short half-life opioid drug, physical stimulation may be enough to prevent significant hypoventilation. No patient has succumbed to respiratory depression while awake. However, if an opiate antagonist is required to reverse respiratory depression or coma in a patient who has been using narcotics chronically, a dilute solution of naloxone should be used (0.4 mg in 10 cc saline-administered as 0.5 cc by i.v. push every two minutes). The dose should be titrated to avoid precipitation of profound withdrawal, seizures, and severe pain. Prior to naloxone administration in a comatose patient, an endotracheal tube should be placed to prevent pulmonary aspiration. In patients receiving meperidine chronically, *naloxone is contraindicated* since it may precipitate seizures by reversing the depressant actions of meperidine, thus allowing the convulsant activity of the active metabolite normeperidine to become evident [28].

Psychological dependence (addiction) is defined as a pattern of compulsive drug use characterized by a continued craving for a narcotic and the need to use the narcotic for effects other than pain relief. The patient exhibits drug-seeking behavior, leading to overwhelming involvement with the use and procurement of the drug. Although most patients with psychological dependence are also physically dependent, the reverse is rarely the case in patients using narcotics for management of pain. The available data suggests that the risk of iatrogenic addiction is very small [29,44,45], and the fear of narcotic addiction should not be a primary concern to the physician in cancer patients. Drug use alone is not the major factor in the development of psychological dependence; other medical, social and economic factors appear to play a more important role [41].

Reasons for choosing a narcotic analgesic in preference to morphine

All narcotics provide similar qualities of analgesia, and as a class, they have similar qualities and frequency of side effects as well. However, individual therapeutic and toxic responses to specific narcotics will vary. Reasons for selecting a narcotic analgesic in preference to morphine (which is the standard against which all others are compared) include the following:

1) A different time-action for analgesia is required. For example, methadone and levorphanol have much longer elimination half-lives (18–24 and 24–36 hours respectively) than morphine (two to three hours), and may provide a slightly longer duration of analgesia than morphine, especially in the opioid-naive patient. Methadone and/or levorphanol should be given every four to six hours to obtain constant pain relief, since the analgesic duration of action is shorter than the plasma half-life.

2) Avoiding a limiting adverse effect of morphine. For example, nausea may be associated with any of the narcotics, but some patients may be more sensitive to the emetic effects of morphine than other narcotics or vice-versa.

3) Taking advantage of incomplete cross-tolerance among the morphinelike drugs by switching to another drug at an equianalgesic dose (see tables 2-1 and 2-2).

4) The availability of a more desirable dosage form:

– *high-potency preparation*: hydromorphone-HP (10 mg/ml) is particularly useful for repetitive subcutaneous or intramuscular injections in an emaciated patient in whom administration of a potent analgesic in limited volume is desirable;

– *rectal suppositories*: hydromorphone (4 mg), numorphan (5 mg), and morphine (5, 10, 20 mg) may be used in patients who cannot take oral drugs because of sedation, confusion, gastrointestinal obstruction, or when s.c. or i.v. administration is impractical.

– *sustained-release morphine preparations*: MS-Contin® and Roxinol-SR® are morphine formulations that are available as 30 mg tablets and have a duration of action of 8–12 hours. The major indication for their use is to provide a longer duration of pain relief, especially at night. Their use may increase patient compliance (since fewer doses need be taken during the day), and they often allow patients to sleep through the night without having to awake to take pain medications. To start a patient on a sustained-release morphine preparation, the 24-hour dose of an *immediate-release* opioid preparation should be calculated (in morphine-equivalents using relative potency estimates given in tables 2-1 and 2-2), and one third or one half of this dose should be given q8–12 hours, respectively, in the sustained-release morphine preparation. If the patient has breakthrough pain, and rescue doses of narcotics are required before the scheduled 8–12 hours, these should be given as required with a standard morphine preparation. Ordinarily, analgesic therapy should not be initiated with sustained release morphine since it is difficult to titrate the patient to optimal pain relief without adverse side effects (especially sedation).

5) When more rapid onset of action is desired. Theoretically, lipophilic drugs such as methadone, meperidine, or fentanyl may be desirable when premedicating a patient for a radiographic or surgical procedure. These drugs have more rapid entry into the brain than morphine and have a faster onset of action.

6) A favorable prior experience with another drug.

Novel routes of opioid administration

Administration of opioids by means other than oral ingestion or intermittent subcutaneous or intravenous injection may be necessary when these routes are impractical or in order to minimize side effects, to provide a more rapid onset and a longer duration of action, or to facilitate nursing care and provide smoother pain control. Guidelines have been published recently for the use of subcutaneous and intravenous infusions of opioids [12,20,37,38,39,46] and there is now nearly a 10-year experience with spinal opioid administration [7,11,43]. Although the safety of these routes of administration has been demonstrated, their use requires sound knowledge of the clinical pharmacology of opioid analgesics and should only be undertaken if patients can be monitored carefully, particularly when used outside of the hospital. In addition, careful clinical studies documenting the efficacy of these routes have been sparse. Therefore, these routes of administration should not be used as first-line treatment for most cancer-related pain, but only in carefully selected patients.

Sublingual administration of opioids may be desirable in patients with bowel obstruction who cannot absorb oral drugs; this route also avoids the first-pass metabolism effect when narcotics are absorbed through the bowel wall. Currently, there are no formulations of narcotic analgesics approved for sublingual administration in the U.S.A., although buprenorphine (Temgesic®) is available in Europe (see table 2-2).

Continuous infusion of narcotics has many advantages over repetitive injections: 1) it avoids delay in the patient receiving injections from the nursing staff and stops clock-watching and other potentially adverse pain behaviors, and 2) it potentially provides smoother pain control by avoiding side effects (at peak plasma drug concentrations) and pain breakthrough (at trough plasma drug concentrations) that can occur with intermittent injections.

Intravenous (i.v.) infusion of opioids is indicated when 1) patients require injections more frequently than every three hours; 2) patients experience prominent bolus effects such as sedation and a rapid return of pain following single injections; or 3) rapid titration of drug is required to produce prompt pain relief [20,38,46]. In a recent study of 36 patients maintained on a total of 46 continuous i.v. infusions from one to 45 days, 28 patients reported "acceptable" pain relief [46]. The range of morphine doses was 0.7–480 mg/hr (mean 52 mg/hr at termination of the infusion), and there were few adverse effects other than sedation, which was reported in 32 of 36 patients [46]. These authors documented that continuous infusion of a variety of narcotics is efficacious in selected patients, and reported a series of guidelines for the selection of patients, the selection of starting and maintenance doses, and the safe use of this technique [46]. It is suggested that repetitive i.v. injections precede initiation of continuous infusion to provide some estimate of dose requirements for individual patients.

Subcutaneous infusion obviates the need for intravenous access and allows long-term parenteral administration of opioids outside of the hospital [8,12,37,39,56]. The indications for its use are similar to intravenous infusion, and this route is particularly effective and useful in children and emaciated patients who require prolonged administration of parenteral narcotics and in whom loss of subcutaneous and muscle bulk makes repetitive injections painful. In addition, Ventrafridda has reported that nausea, vomiting, and constipation occur less commonly with continuous subcutaneous infusion in comparison to oral administration [56]. Plasma morphine levels are similar when subcutaneous infusions are compared to intravenous infusions at 24 hours [57]. Any opioid may be infused by the subcutaneous or intravenous routes, but it is perhaps best to use short half-life drugs (such as morphine or hydromorphone) since dose titration is easier because drug accumulation over time is less dramatic than with long half-life drugs. Infusions of meperidine should be avoided since it is irritating to tissues and may be associated with the accumulation of normeperidine with resultant tremors, multifocal myoclonus, and seizures.

In a recent series, 13 of 15 adult cancer patients treated with continuous s.c. infusion of narcotics for three to 76 days reported "satisfactory" pain relief [12]. Nine patients in this series were given continuous morphine infusions in doses ranging from 3.5–97.0 mg/hr [12]. In children, morphine doses of 0.025–0.09 mg/kg/hr have been reported [39]. Infusion of drugs is accomplished with a portable infusion pump connected to a 27-gauge butterfly needle inserted subcutaneously. Guidelines for use of this technique have been published [12].

Patient-controlled analgesia involves the intermittent bolus administration of opioids, the frequency of administration being determined by the patient. This is usually accomplished with a drug delivery device in which the physician can program the dose or infusion rate and maximum frequency of drug injection available to the patient. By pushing a button, the patient can decide on the timing of a preselected dose, volume, and/or concentration of drug to be delivered by the intravenous, subcutaneous, or epidural route of administration. Patient-controlled analgesia has been studied most extensively by the intravenous route in the management of post-operative pain [21,52]. Current data suggest that patients will titrate the frequency of administration to maintain a minimally effective plasma concentration with minimum side effects without overdosing themselves, and when offered a choice, prefer this method to more conventional methods of postoperative pain management. Patient-controlled analgesia may also have a role in the management of incident pain secondary to tumor metastasis in bone and peripheral nerve, since the patient can administer a dose of medication in anticipation of movement.

Spinal epidural or subarachnoid (intrathecal) administration may be accomplished by intermittent injection through reservoir devices or by continuous infusion through implantable and external pumps. Spinal opioids have the potential advantage of affording long durations of pain relief (18 hours or longer) after administration of small doses (5–10 mg morphine) in comparison to intravenous or subcutaneous administration [7,11,43]. The indications for spinal opiate administration in cancer pain are still being defined, but this route may be particularly useful in patients with bilateral or midline pain (of somatic or visceral origin) below the umbilicus, in whom adequate pain relief cannot be obtained with systemic opioids because of doselimiting side effects [1,43]. Epidural or intrathecal morphine administration is associated with significant levels of drug in the plasma, however, and bloodborne drug delivery to the brain, coupled with rostral CSF redistribution of drug, may produce nausea and vomiting, sedation, and respiratory depression [9,11,36,43]. All patients should undergo myelography prior to initiation of spinal opiate therapy, since obstruction of the epidural or subarachnoid space by tumor metastasis is frequent in cancer patients and is a major contraindication to the use of this technique. Spinal opiate administration shows cross-tolerance with systemically administered opiates, and may be associated with the need for rapid dose escalation with chronic use [22]. The rapid development of tolerance that may occur with spinal opiate administration has been a major limiting feature [36,43].

Intraventricular morphine administration has been used to manage head and neck pain and diffuse pain caused by advanced metastatic cancer [32,33,35,47]. Lobato reported that 81% of 44 patients reported "excellent" pain relief lasting an average 22 hours after 0.5 or 1.0 mg injection of morphine into a subcutaneous reservoir connected to the lateral cerebral ventricle [35]. The onset of pain relief occurred within an average of 15 minutes after injection. Thirty percent of the patients in this series experienced side effects such as nausea, vomiting, pruritus, urinary retention and sedation [35]. Although profound analgesia may be achieved with smaller doses of drug than would be required with systemic administration, the advantage of intraventricular narcotic administration over more conventional routes is still unclarified. In particular, the rate of development of tolerance to repetitive intraventricular administration is not clear.

Potentially hazardous narcotics

Pentazocine is the only mixed agonist–antagonist narcotic analgesic available in an oral formulation (table 2-3). The mixed agonist–antagonist drugs bind to opioid receptors to produce analgesia (and are, therefore, opioid agonists), but also have antagonist properties—they reverse opioid analgesia and can precipitate withdrawal when given to patients who are taking morphinelike agonists. Pentazocine may cause confusion and hallucinations, particularly when dose escalations are required to manage severe pain [6]. For these reasons and others, the routine use of pentazocine cannot be recommended for management of cancer pain.

Meperidine is a synthetic, short-acting narcotic (three to four hours) with poor oral potency (300 mg p.o. is roughly equivalent to 10 mg of i.m. morphine in single-dose analgesic studies). Normeperidine, a metabolite of meperidine, is a central nervous system stimulant and will produce anxiety, tremors, myoclonus, and generalized seizures if it accumulates with repetitive dosing of meperidine [28]. This is more likely to occur in patients with compromised renal function [28]. The hyperexcitability is not reversed with naloxone, and in fact, the administration of naloxone to patients receiving meperidine chronically may precipitate seizures [28]. For these reasons, meperidine should not be used chronically.

ADJUVANT ANALGESICS (see table 2-3)

These agents may be useful when combined with narcotic or nonnarcotic analgesics [18]. In some neuropathic pain syndromes, they are the drug of choice [18,51]. The classes of drugs that are used as adjuvant analgesics are as follows.

Table 2-3. Adjuvant analgesic drugs useful in cancer pain management

Drug	Usual Dose and Route of Administration	Indications for Use	Comment
Amitriptyline (Elavil®, others)	10–125 mg p.o./day 2–5 mg/kg/day[a]	Deafferentation pain	Start treatment at 10 mg HS for elderly (25 mg HS for others) and slowly escalate to 125 mg as tolerated over 1–2 weeks. *Side Effects:* sedation, dry mouth, urinary retention (esp. in elderly males)
Fluphenazine (Prolixin®, others)	1–3 mg p.o./day .02–.05 mg/kg/dose[a] to 1 mg/8hr	Deafferentation pain	Usually used in combination with amitriptyline (50–100 mg) or imipramine (50–100 mg). *Side Effects:* sedation, orthostatic hypotension, extrapyramidal effects, including tardive dyskinesia
Methotrimeprazine (Levoprome®)	10–15 mg I.M.; then 10–20 mg I.M. q6–8h	Opioid tolerant patients; to avoid severe opioid-induced constipation or respiratory depression	Not available orally. Should give 10–15 mg I.M. test dose. Analgesic effects are independent of opioid effects. 15 mg I.M. equipotent to 15 mg I.M. morphine. *Side Effects:* orthostatic hypotension, sedation, extrapyramidal effects, including tardive dyskinesia
Haloperidol (Haldol®)	0.5–1.0 mg p.o. BID or TID .05–.075 mg/kg/day[a]	Coanalgesic (with opioids) in acutely agitated or psychotic patients	May potentiate morphine analgesia, and allow reduction in dose. Antipsychotic dose is higher (10 mg BID or TID). *Side Effects:* sedation, hypotension, extrapyramidal effects, including tardive dyskinesia
Dextroamphetamine (Dexedrine®)	5–10 mg p.o. BID 2–10 mg/day[a]	Reduce sedative effects of narcotics	Avoid giving last dose in evening to minimize insomnia. May be coanalgesic with morphine in postoperative pain management. *Side Effects:* tachycardia, agitation, insomnia

Drug	Dose	Indication	Comments
Dexamethasone (Decadron®)	4–8 mg p.o. QID	Refractory bone and deafferentation pain. Epidural spinal cord compression (ESCC)	May have specific oncolytic effects. Dose and route of administration vary depending on clinical situation (may give up to 100 mg I.V. bolus for acute ESCC). Usually give over 1–2 week period. May give equivalent in Prednisone *Side Effects* (with acute use): weight gain, G.I. hemorrhaging, myopathy, psychosis (rare). Avoid concomitant NSAID use
Carbamazepine (Tegretol®)	200 mg/day (start) 800–1200 mg/day	Deafferentation pain (esp. with lancinating or shooting qualities)	Should check blood counts at regular intervals. *Side Effects:* nausea, dizziness, ataxia
Hydroxyzine (Vistaril®, others)	25–50 mg p.o./i.m. q6h 0.2–0.5 mg/kg/day[a]	Coanalgesic in anxious, nauseated patient	Synergistic analgesic effect with narcotics. *Side Effect:* drowsiness

[a] Pediatric Dose Ranges—see Reference 49.
Adapted from Payne R (1987): Pain. In: Wittes RE (ed), *Manual of Oncologic Therapeutics*. Philadelphia: J.B. Lippincott Co.

Anticonvulsants (phenytoin, carbamazepine)

These are particularly useful for the management of pain in chronic neuralgias such as trigeminal neuralgia, postherpetic neuralgia, glossopharyngeal neuralgia, and posttraumatic neuralgias. These neuralgias may complicate tumor progression (i.e., glossopharyngeal neuralgia in head and neck cancers) or cancer therapy (i.e., intercostal neuralgia secondary to thoracotomy). Carbamazepine (400–800 mg/ day or higher) is the drug of choice for management of any painful peripheral neuropathy in which there is a paroxysmal, shooting electric shocklike quality to the pain [18]. It is generally less useful in managing the burning and aching sensations associated with neuropathic pain.

Phenothiazines (methotrimeprazine, fluphenazine)

Methotrimeprazine (Levoprome 20 mg/cc; available in parenteral formulation only) provides pain relief by a nonopioid mechanism [3]; it may be useful for the treatment of opioid-tolerant patients and to avoid the constipating and respiratory-depressant effects of narcotics, but sedation and orthostatic hypotension are limiting side effects [3,18]. Fluphenazine is also a useful adjuvant analgesic, particularly when used in combination with a tricyclic antidepressant (i.e., imipramine or amitriptyline) [18]. All phenothiazines are useful to combat narcotic-induced emesis. They are not used routinely in combination with narcotics because they may exacerbate the sedative effects of narcotics.·

Tricyclic antidepressants (amitriptyline, imipramine, doxepin)

These agents provide direct analgesic effects, possibly through their action of blocking the re-uptake of serotonin and norepinephrine at CNS synapses [5,13,50]. Amitriptyline has the best-documented analgesic actions [58], but is also the least well-tolerated because of its potent anticholinergic effects (dry mouth, urinary retention, delirium). Sedation and orthostatic hypotension may also be limiting side effects in the use of tricyclic compounds. The analgesic effects are seen at lower doses (typically 25–150 mg/day for amitriptyline) than are their antidepressant effects. These drugs may ameliorate insomnia and may be given at bedtime for this additional beneficial effect. Their use is recommended for a wide variety of cancer pain syndromes including pain associated with terminal illness [13] and, in particular, pain due to peripheral nerve injury such as postherpetic neuralgia, vincristine and cisplatin-induced neuropathy, and postthoracotomy or postlaparotomy incisional pain.

Dextroamphetamine

Dextroamphetamine may produce additive analgesia when combined with narcotics in the postoperative period [19]. An additional indication for its use is the reduction of sedative effects of narcotics in cancer patients who are not able to function, despite adequate pain relief, because of sedation.

Steroids

Steroids have specific and nonspecific effects in managing acute and chronic cancer pain. They may be oncolytic for some tumors (e.g., lymphoma) and may ameliorate painful nerve or spinal cord compression by reducing edema in tumor and nervous tissue. Their use is standard emergency practice in the treatment of suspected malignant spinal cord compression (dexamethasone 16–96 mg/day or its equivalent). One to two weeks of steroid treatment may be useful in management of pain caused by malignant lesions of the brachial or lumbosacral plexus in patients in whom large doses of opioids are ineffective. In the moribund patient, steroids may provide euphoria and increase the appetite as well as relieve tumor-related pain; chronic side effects are not to be feared in this situation.

Chronic use produces weight gain, Cushing's syndrome, proximal myopathy, psychosis (rarely), and increases the risk of G.I. bleeding (especially when used in combination with NSAIDs). In addition, rapid withdrawal of steroids may exacerbate pain independent of progression of systemic cancer (pseudorheumatoid syndrome) [48].

Antihistamines

Hydroxyzine has analgesic and antiemetic activity in addition to its antihistamine effects. The usual dose is 25–50 mg p.o./i.m. q6 hours prn. It may produce additive analgesia when combined with narcotics, with only slightly more sedation, so that it is a useful adjuvant for the anxious, nauseated patient [2].

Agents to be avoided

Benzodiazepines are effecive for treatment of acute anxiety attacks and muscle spasm, but do not have analgesic or co-analgesic properties. Their routine use is not recommended for the treatment of chronic cancer pain. Although acute pain is often associated with typical signs of anxiety, treatment should focus on the cause of pain and the use of specific analgesic agents; benzodiazepines are not indicated.

Sedative-hypnotic drugs (i.e., barbiturates) do not have intrinsic analgesic properties and should generally be avoided in the management of pain. Many commonly used analgesics are formulated in combination with barbiturates (Belladenal®, Fiorinal®, Axotal®) and must be prescribed with caution.

Cannabinoids Although delta-9 tetrahydrocannabinol (THC) has been shown to have analgesic properties in controlled clinical studies [23], it is associated with high incidence of dysphoria, drowsiness, hypotension, and bradycardia. Its routine use cannot be recommended for management of pain in cancer, although it does have some efficacy as an antiemetic for chemotherapy-induced nausea and vomiting.

Cocaine has local anesthetic properties, but controlled trials have demonstrated no efficacy as an analgesic or co-analgesic in combination with narcotics [53].

COMMON MISCONCEPTIONS REGARDING DRUG THERAPY IN CANCER PAIN

Placebo response

The placebo response is a common occurrence in patients. A positive analgesic effect from i.m. saline does not provide any useful information about the genesis or severity of the pain. In fact, many patients who have a documented organic basis for their pain obtain some temporary relief when given a placebo. The deceptive use of placebos and the misinterpretation of the placebo response to distinguish psycho-genic from real pain should be avoided.

Pain in children

Children may have acute or chronic pain, but inadequate verbal skills and/or their misconceptions about the etiology or consequences of pain may alter the symptoms and signs. For example, children may not report pain because they fear it will lead to painful diagnostic evaluations. An abnormal gait, failure to move an extremity, or persistent crying may be the only clue to the existence of pain. In practice, alterations in heart rate and blood pressure in acute pain or changes in activity levels in acute and chronic pain are the best assessments of pain in children. The assessment of pain in preverbal children is particularly difficult. These children should receive narcotic analgesics when noxious stimuli are produced by surgical procedures.

Young children may refuse to take oral medication or intermittent injections. Therefore, the intravenous route is used in the majority of children who cannot, or will not, take oral medications. Narcotic infusions are indicated when pain control is unsatisfactory using intermittent narcotic dosing; continuous intravenous or sub-cutaneous infusions (using a portable syringe pump) have been found to yield adequate pain relief in the majority of these patients.

In choosing the starting dose of narcotic analgesics for children for management of postoperative or cancer pain, the age, weight, and prior narcotic experience of the child should be considered [49]. It is generally recommended that children 12 years of age and older require full adult doses (using 10 mg morphine i.m. as the standard dose as depicted in tables 2-2 and 2-3). Children seven to 12 years old generally require 50% of the starting adult dose and children two to six years of age require 20–25% of the starting adult dose. For infants under two years of age, the starting morphine dose is generally 0.1–0.2 mg/kg/dose i.v. or 0.5–1.2 mg/kg/dose p.o. [49]. It must be emphasized that these are starting doses, and as in the adult patient, dose titration up or down is always necessary to obtain analgesia with a minimum of side effects. There is no evidence that preadolescent and adolescent children are at higher risk for addiction than the general population when narcotics are prescribed for the management of pain. Like adults, they will develop tolerance during chronic narcotic treatment and may require larger doses to adequately control their pain, especially children with advanced cancer.

Use of analgesics in the elderly

Analgesics may be given safely to geriatric patients, although adjustments of doses are usually required [27]. For example, plasma levels of tricyclic compounds are usually higher, for a given dose, in older as compared to younger patients [40]. Intramuscular morphine produces a longer duration of analgesia in older patients, in part related to prolonged elimination from blood in the elderly [27]. In addition, elderly as well as younger patients with central nervous system disease may be more sensitive to opioids. Therefore, the titration of analgesic dose to a given response is even more critical in these patients.

Heroin and cancer pain

Although oral or parenteral diacetylmorphine (heroin) provides pain relief in cancer patients [26,54], it does not offer any unique pharmacokinetic or pharmacodynamic advantages over morphine or other more easily available narcotics for the management of pain of malignant origin [25,26]. Although more soluble than morphine, and thus easier to formulate in more concentrated solutions for parenteral injections, this advantage is no longer important with the availability of a high-potency hydromorphone preparation (Dilaudid-HP, 10 mg/ml) that is even more potent than heroin. The effects of heroin are due to its in vivo biotransformation to morphine and perhaps 6-acetylmorphine [25].

SUMMARY OF CLINICAL APPROACH TO MANAGEMENT OF CANCER PAIN WITH ANALGESICS

The following is a stepwise clinical approach to drug treatment of patients with acute or chronic cancer-related pain [16,17,24].

1. Start with a nonnarcotic analgesic (e.g., aspirin 650 mg or its equivalent every four to six hours). These agents may be effective without producing tolerance or physical dependence. The use of all aspirinlike drugs except choline magnesium salicylate and acetaminophen may be limited in the thrombocytopenic or surgical patient due to their antiplatelet effects and G.I. toxicity. The nonnarcotic analgesics have a ceiling effect; for aspirin this is roughly 1000 mg/day. Increasing the dose beyond this amount may increase the duration of analgesia, but will not increase the peak effect.

2. If additional analgesia is required, add a weak narcotic agonist such as oxycodone or codeine. (See tables 2-2 and 2-3 for typical starting doses.) Oxycodone and codeine have no ceiling effect, but dose escalation is frequently limited by side effects such as nausea and mental clouding.

3. If more analgesia is required, then switch to a stronger narcotic (methadone, levorphanol, morphine, hydromorphone; see tables 2-2 and 2-3 for typical starting doses). Although they are strong narcotics, morphine and hydromorphone have short durations of effect (three to four hours). Levorphanol and methadone will accumulate with repetitive dosing, reaching steady-state after five to six half-lives (two to three days for levorphanol; five to six days for methadone).

4. Beware that in switching from a short half-life drug (e.g., morphine or hydromorphone) to a long half-life drug (e.g., levorphanol or methadone), a reduction in dose may be needed after 24 hours; the long half-life drug progressively accumulates over the first three to five days of therapy. Conversely, in switching from a long to short half-life drug, increased doses may be needed as early as 12 hours as the former drug is eliminated from the body over three to five days.

5. Use adjuvant drugs to enhance the therapeutic effects and counteract the adverse effects of narcotics. For neuropathic pain, amitriptyline and carbamazepine (if pain is shooting in quality) may be drugs of choice.

6. Respect individual differences among patients and expect to titrate the dose of

analgesics to maximum effect. Ask the patient if pain relief is adequate so that you can rapidly adjust the dose if necessary. Otherwise, patients may put up with suboptimal doses of analgesics, particularly if they (inappropriately) fear that addiction will occur as a result of chronic use.

ACKNOWLEDGMENTS

The author is a recipient of a Robert Wood Johnson Minority Faculty Development Award, and a grant from the National Cancer Institute CA 32897-03S1. The author wishes to thank Dr. Mitchell Max for his comments and criticisms of this manuscript, and Marilyn Herleth for preparation of this manuscript. Relative potency ratios are derived from the work of Dr. Raymond Houde, and tables 2-1 and 2-2 were written in collaboration with Dr. Charles E. Inturrisi.

REFERENCES

1. Arner S, Arner B (1985): Differential effects of epidural morphine in the treatment of cancer-related pain. Acta Anaesthesiol Scand 29:32–36.
2. Beaver WT, Feise G (1976): Comparison of the analgesic effects of morphine, hydroxyzine and their combination in patients with post-operative pain. In: Bonica JJ, Albe-Fessard D (eds), Advances in Pain Research and Therapy. New York: Raven Press, pp 553–557.
3. Beaver WT, Wallenstein SL, Houde RW, et al. (1966): A comparison of the analgesic effect of methotrimeprazine and morphine in patients with cancer. Clin Pharmacol Ther 7:436–446.
4. Bonica, JJ (1985): The treatment of cancer pain: current status and future needs. In: Fields HL et al. (eds), Advances in Pain Research and Therapy, vol 9. New York: Raven Press, pp 589–616.
5. Botney M, Fields HL (1983): Amitriptyline potentiates morphine analgesia by a direct action on the central nervous system. Ann Neurol 13:160–164.
6. Brogden RN, Speigt TM, Avery GS (1973): Pentazocine: a review of pharmacological properties, therapeutics, efficacy and dependence. Drugs 5:6–91.
7. Bromage PR (1985): Clinical aspects of intrathecal and epidural opiates. In: Fields HL et al. (eds), Advances in Pain Research and Therapy, vol 9. New York: Raven Press, pp 733–748.
8. Campbell CF, Matson JB, Weiler JM (1983): Continuous subcutaneous infusion of morphine for the pain of terminal malignancy. Ann Int Med 98:51–52.
9. Chauvin M, Samii K, Schermann JM, et al. (1982): Plasma pharmacokinetics of morphine after i.m., extradural and intrathecal administration. Br J Anaesth 54:843–848.
10. Cleeland CS, Cleeland LM, Dar R, et al. (1986): Factors in influencing physician management of cancer pain. Cancer 58:796–800.
11. Cousins MJ, Mather LE (1984): Intrathecal and epidural administration of opioids. Anesthesiology 61:276–310.
12. Coyle N, Mauskop A, Maggard J, et al. (1986): Continuous subcutaneous infusion of opiates in cancer patients with pain. Onc Nurs Forum 13:53–57.
13. Feinmann C (1985): Pain relief by antidepressants: possible modes of action. Pain 23:1–8.
14. Foley, KM (1981): Current issues in the management of cancer pain: Memorial Sloan-Kettering Cancer Center. In: Loreng NG (ed), New Approaches to Treatment of Chronic Pain. Nida Research Monograph 36:169–181.
15. Foley KM (1982): The practical use of narcotic analgesics. Med Clin North Am 66:1091–1104.
16. Foley, KM, Sundaresan N (1984): Management of cancer pain. In: Devita VT, Hellman S, Rosenberg SA (eds), Cancer: Principles and Practice of Oncology. Philadelphia: J.B. Lippincott Co., pp 1941–1961.
17. Foley KM (1985): The treatment of cancer pain. N Engl J Med 313:84–95.
18. Foley KM (1985): Adjuvant analgesic drugs in cancer pain management. In: Aronoff GM (ed), Evaluation and Treatment of Chronic Pain. Baltimore-Munich: Urban and Schwarzenberg.
19. Forrest WH, Brown BW, Brown CR, et al. (1977): Dextroamphetamine with morphine for the treatment of postoperative pain. N Engl J Med 296:712–715.
20. Fraser DG (1980): Intravenous morphine infusion for chronic pain. Ann Int Med 93:781–782.

21. Graves D, Foster TS, Batenhorst RL, et al. (1983): Patient-controlled analgesia. Ann Int Med 99:360–366.
22. Greenberg HS, Taren J, Ensminger WD, Doan K (1982): Benefit from and tolerance to containuous intrathecal infusion of morphine for intractable cancer pain. J Neurosurg 57:360–364.
23. Harris LS (1979): Cannabinoids as analgesics. In: Beers RF, Bassett EG (eds), New York: Raven Press. Mechanism of Pain and Analgesic Compounds.
24. Houde RW (1974): The use and misuse of narcotics in the treatment of chronic pain. Adv Neurol 4:527–536.
25. Inturrisi CE, Max MB, Foley KM, et al. (1984): The pharmacokinetics of heroin in patients with chronic pain. N Engl J Med 210:1213–1217.
26. Kaiko RF, Wallenstein SL, Rogers AG, et al. (1981): Analgesic and mood effects of heroin and morphine in cancer patients with postoperative pain. N Engl J Med 304:1501–1505.
27. Kaiko RF, Wallenstein SL, Rogers AG, et al. (1982): Narcotics in the elderly. Med Clin North Am 66:1079–1089.
28. Kaiko RF, Foley KM, Grabinski PY, et al. (1983): Central nervous system excitatory effects of meperidine in cancer patients. Ann Neurol 13:180–185.
29. Kanner RM, Foley KM (1981): Patterns of narcotic drug use in a cancer pain clinic. Ann NY Acad Sci 362:161–172.
30. Kantor TG (1982): The control of pain by nonsteroidal anti-inflammatory drugs. Med Clin North Am 66:1053–1059.
31. King JS, Gallant P, Myerson V, et al. (1976): The effects of anti-inflammatory agents on the responses and the sensitization of unmyelinated (C) fiber polymodal receptors. In: Zotterman Y (ed), Sensory Function of the Skin of Primates. Oxford: Pergamon Press, pp 441–461.
32. Leavens ME, Hill CS, Cech DA, et al. (1982): Intrathecal and intraventricular morphine for pain in cancer patients: initial study. J Neurosurg 56:241–242.
33. Lenzi A, Galli G, Gandolfini M, et al. (1985): Intraventricular morphine in paraneoplastic painful syndrome of the cervicofacial region: experience in thirty-eight cases. Neurosurgery 17:6–11.
34. Levin D, Cleeland CS, Dar R (1985): Public attitudes toward cancer pain. Cancer 56:2337–2339.
35. Lobato RD, Madrid JL, Fatela LV, et al. (1985): Analgesia elicited by low-dose intraventricular morphine in terminal cancer patients. In: Fields HL et al. (eds), Advances in Pain Research and Therapy, vol 9. New York: Raven Press, pp 673–681.
36. Max MB, Inturrisi CE, Kaiko RF, et al. (1985): Epidural and intrathecal opiates: cerebrospinal fluid and plasma profiles in patients with chronic cancer pain. Clin Pharmacol Ther 38:631–641.
37. Miser AW, Davis DM, Hughes CS, et al. (1983): Continuous subcutaneous infusions of morphine in children with cancer. Am J Dis Child 137:383–385.
38. Miser AW, Miser JS, Clark BS (1980): Continuous intravenous infusion of morphine sulfate for control of severe pain in children with terminal malignancy. J Pediatr 5:930–932.
39. Nahata MC, Miser AW, Miser JS, et al. (1984): Analgesic plasma concentrations of morphine in children with terminal malignancy receiving a continuous subcutaneous infusion of morphine sulfate to control severe pain. Pain 18:109–114.
40. Neis A, Robinson DS, Friedman MJ, et al. (1977): Relationship between age and tricyclic antidepressant plasma levels. Am J Psychiat 134:790–793.
41. Newman RG (1983): The need to redefine "addiction". N Engl J Med 308:1096–1098.
42. Payne R, Foley KM (1984): Advances in the management of cancer pain. Cancer Treat Rep 68:173–83.
43. Payne R (1986): The role of spinal opiates and opioid peptides in the management of cancer pain. Med Clin North Am (in press).
44. Perry S, Heidrich G (1982): Management of pain during debridement: a survey of U.S. burn units. Pain 13:267–280.
45. Porter J, Jick H (1980): Addiction rare in patients treated with narcotics. N Engl J Med 302:133.
46. Portenoy RK, Moulin DE, Rogers A, et al. (1986): I.V. infusion of opioids for cancer pain: clinical review and guidelines for use. Cancer Treat Rep 70:575–581.
47. Roquefeuil B, Benezech J, Blanchet P, et al. (1984): Intraventricular administration of morphine in patients with neoplastic intractable pain. Surg Neurol 21:155–158.
48. Rotstein J, Good RA (1957): Steroid pseudorheumatism. Arch Int Med 99:545–555.
49. Schlechter NE (1985): Pain and pain control in children. Curr Prob Pediatr 15:1–67.
50. Spiegel K, Kalb R, Pasternak GW (1983): Analgesic activity of tricyclic antidepressants. Ann Neurol 13:462–465.
51. Swerdlow M (1984): Anticonvulsant drugs and chronic pain. Clin Neuropharmacol 7:51–82.

52. Tameson A, Hartvig P, Fagerlund C, et al. (1982): Patient-controlled analgesia: clinical experience. Acta Anesthesiol Scand (Suppl) 14:157–160.
53. Twycross RG (1977): Value of cocaine in opiate-containing elixirs. Br Med J 2:1348.
54. Twycross RG (1977): Choice of strong analgesic in terminal cancer: diamorphine or morphine? Pain 3:93–104.
55. Twycross RG, Lack SA (1983): Symptom Control in Far Advanced Cancer: Pain Relief. London: Pitman Publishing.
56. Ventafridda V, Spoldi E, Caraceni A, et al. (1986): The importance of continuous subcutaneous morphine administration for cancer pain. The Pain Clinic 1:47–55.
57. Waldmann CS, Eason JR, Rambohul E, et al. (1984): Serum morphine levels. A comparison between continuous subcutaneous infusion and continuous intravenous infusion in postoperative patients. Anaesthesia 39:768–771.
58. Watson CP, Evans RJ, Reid K, et al. (1982): Amitriptyline vs. placebo in postherpetic neuralgia. Neurology 32:671–73.

3. PSYCHOLOGICAL ASPECTS OF PAIN DUE TO CANCER

CHARLES S. CLEELAND, PH.D.

Pain is a major component of the cancer patient's suffering. Unrelieved pain can lead to a resignation to death, even before curative efforts for the disease have been exhausted. It is a never-ending reminder of the gravity of the disease and its progression. Severe pain can divert the attention that needs to be paid to family, friends, and the effort of coming to terms with death. Pain also contributes to loss of sleep, appetite, and a reduction of activity, and thus increases impairment directly measurable in indices of disease status [1].

It is not surprising that pain is one of the most feared aspects of having cancer. In a survey of public attitudes toward cancer pain, an interview-based study found that cancer was rated significantly more painful than several other medical conditions, with the exception of migraine headache and heart attack [2]. Approximately half of this sample rated cancer as very or extremely painful. Almost two thirds agreed with the opinion that cancer pain can become so severe that patients would consider abandoning life-prolonging treatment, or even consider suicide. Cancer *treatment* was also considered to be very or extremely painful by 42% of the respondents, with another 37% viewing treatment as moderately painful. Eighteen percent agreed that they would avoid seeking care for cancer because of the fear of the pain associated with treatment.

Having to be treated for cancer pain can also provoke anxiety. The sample was asked to rate their concerns about taking analgesics for pain due to cancer. About half of all respondents had significant concerns about taking potent analgesics, including confusion and disorientation, developing tolerance to the effectiveness of the drugs the risk of addiction, and suffering from other negative side effects.

Given this matrix of public perception, it is not surprising that cancer patients, once receiving their diagnosis, are anxious about the pain that they expect they will have to endure. They will fear that their disease will cause additional pain. They will associate the presence of pain with worsening of their disease. Furthermore, they will anticipate that having to take potent analgesics for pain will put them at risk for addiction and additional negative side effects.

PAIN AND MOOD DISTURBANCES

Once pain is present, cancer patients will be at greater risk for depression and other types of mood disturbance. In a study where cancer patients with pain were matched with patients who had similar disease status but were without pain, the patients with pain obtained higher scores on measures of depression as well as measures of anxiety, hostility, and somatization. Those with pain were also less active [3].

Are those patients who are already depressed at higher risk for pain? Some reports suggest that measures of mood disturbance are predictive of the severity of pain later in the course of the disease [4]. Noting that patients with severe pain report more neuroticism, Bond [5] suggested that there may be a common neurophysiologic mechanism shared by pain and emotional disturbance. He acknowledged, however, that emotional disturbance may be due to the presence of pain, and that the cancer pain patients he studied had less evidence of emotional disturbance than a comparison group of patients with other medical conditions. He also noted a reduction in neuroticism among patients who obtained pain relief from treatment.

An example of the difficulty in sorting out the relationship between pain and depression is illustrated in a report by Spiegel and Bloom [6]. They studied 86 women with carcinoma of the breast, 56% of whom reported pain. They obtained measures of mood, coping response, analgesic use, and beliefs about the significance of pain. They used a rating of "suffering" as a measure of pain. They concluded that variation in pain, or "suffering," was not primarily due to the physical aspects of the illness itself, but to psychological factors. The authors did qualify their findings, noting that correlational studies do not establish causation. It is important to keep this qualification in mind, since one of their measures of physical contribution was time to death, which may not be correlated with pain in a reasonably homogeneous group of patients with metastatic disease. A better measure would have been to use detailed physical examination of the patient, rating the subjects on who was most likely to have pain based on physical causes. The second problem with this study is that several of their measures of "psychological contribution" (analgesic use, mood scale ratings) are known to be quite reactive to the severity of pain that the patient experiences.

Depression is not a universal accompaniment of cancer. One study of patients hospitalized at a major cancer center found that 24% of cancer patients (both with and without pain) were depressed [7]. This study found that the most physically ill patients tended to be more depressed. Studies comparing cancer patients with patients hospitalized with other medical conditions [8,9] have found that cancer patients were not significantly more depressed than other patients. There is also evidence that not all cancer patients with pain, even those with severe pain, are depressed.

We studied 120 patients with advanced cancer who also had moderate to severe pain [1]. Approximately one third of this group were labeled by at least one member of the treatment team as depressed. Using this very inclusive criterion for depression, we found no difference in pain intensity measures between those who were and those who were not labeled as depressed. As part of this study, patients completed the Brief Symptom Inventory (BSI). Those who scored in the top third of the depression scale of this measure were compared with those who scored in the bottom third. Again, no significant differences were found between the groups on pain intensity ratings. No differences between groups were found in ratings of health status. The depressed group did report that their pain *interfered* more with their mood and activity.

As part of this same project, we examined the relationship between depression and pain in another way. We asked if pain would be less responsive to pain therapy in the more depressed patients. We computed pain change scores for the 115 patients who survived the first month of the study. Depression, as measured by the BSI, was not predictive of pain change. Scales sampling hostility and anxiety were also not associated with pain change. Our findings were consistent with other studies which have failed to find an association between measures of emotional disturbance and response to pain treatment in cancer patients [5,10].

Finally, we studied the relationship between mood and pain in a group of cancer patients with pain who were assessed on five separate occasions one month apart [11]. The relationship between pain measures and mood measures was examined using both individual (cross-sectional) and intraindividual (within-subject) measures of association. Both types of analyses suggested small but significant relationships between pain severity and negative mood, and inverse correlations between measures of positive mood and pain intensity. Despite these relationships, this group of patients with advanced disease and poorly controlled pain reported little mood disturbance on any testing occasion.

To summarize our current understanding of the relationship between cancer pain and mood disturbance, there is evidence that severe pain worsens mood, but not to the extent that would be expected. More depressed patients are likely to report that pain interferes more with activity and mood, but are not likely to report that their pain is more intense. Patients who report more depression on psychometric measures or who appear more depressed to clinicians do not respond less favorably to appropriate pain therapy.

Despite the lack of evidence that depression affects the intensity of a patient's report of pain, many physicians assume that new complaints of pain or complaints of pain no longer relieved by analgesics is a way of expressing emotional distress. In a study of physicians who treat cancer patients [12], we found two groups: one smaller group with more liberal attitudes toward pain management, and a larger group defined as having more typical attitudes toward pain and its management. In the typical group, amost half of the physicians reported that they regarded a new complaint of pain as an expression of anxiety or of depression, rather than as a veridical report of increased pain. This finding is similar to an earlier report [13] that noted that patients were often referred to psychiatry because of suspected depression when the actual problem was undermedication for severe pain.

COMMUNICATION ABOUT PAIN

One way that psychological factors influence the quality of cancer pain management is reflected in the difficulty that physicians and patients have when it comes to open communication about pain and the disruption pain causes in the patient's life. Adequate management of pain and associated distress can only be achieved when the health care team has an accurate picture of the problem. Although some health care staff feel that patients tend to overemphasize distress, the data suggest that patients more often tend to understate the distress that they experience. Patients may underreport pain and distress for many reasons. For example, patients may fear that, if they complain too much about pain or psychological distress, staff will be distracted from the task of curing their disease [14]. This is more likely to happen when staff have limited time to give to each patient, forcing the patient to formulate priorities for the staff time available to them. Other patients feel that their behavior with staff will influence the quality of their care in general. They may feel that good patients will be rewarded by receiving more time from staff. Since patients are not provided with a script for being a good patient, they automatically assume that complaining of pain or distress is not part of the good patient role. For the same reason, patients may be reluctant to tell staff that analgesic therapy is not working. In many instances, their assumptions will be reinforced when they find that busy staff are much more willing to spend time with them when they don't complain. One study has reported that physicians rank patients who complain of unresolved pain among those with whom they least like to spend time [15]. Finally, patients may minimize complaints of pain because they assume that having pain is a natural part of their illness or its treatment and not expect that pain can be managed.

ASSESSMENT OF PAIN AND ITS EFFECTS

A thoughtful assessment strategy can minimize patient reluctance to report pain and its lack of relief, as well as such other associated symptoms of distress as mood and sleep disturbance. At a minimum, the assessment should ask a standard set of questions using a common measurement scale. Several scales for measuring subjective symptoms are available, and they tend to produce equivalent data in clinical practice [16]. Once a metric has been assigned to represent pain severity, the values obtained can be charted for monitoring pain severity and its response to treatment. This record is especially helpful during initial analgesic titration.

Several types of pain severity scales have been proposed, including categorical ("mild" versus "moderate" versus "severe"), visual analogue (where patients respond by marking on a 10-cm line, with the left side signifying "no pain" and the

A. Categorical				
Mild	Moderate	Severe	Horrible	Excruciating

B. Visual analogue
No pain _____ pain as bad as could be

C. Numeric
No pain   0 1 2 3 4 5 6 7 8 9 10   Pain as bad as could be

Figure 3-1. Scales for measuring pan severity. In (A) the patient chooses the word that most describes the severity of pain. In (B) the patient makes a mark to correspond with the *analog* of pain severity, while in (C), the patient rates pain severity by choosing a number of correspond to pain severity.

right side "pain as bad as you can imagine"). Numeric scales, where the patient selects a number representing pain severity, have a practical advantage, because patients easily grasp the idea of how to respond to them and patients can report their symptoms orally when they are unable to write.

Figure 3-1 gives an example of these various scales. While pain-rating scales may be used in the format of a clinical interview, presenting them to the patient in the form of a simple questionnaire has distinct advantages. Patients are often less concerned about responding openly to a questionnaire than to oral questions put to them by staff. Questionnaires never forget to ask all the pertinent questions; they can be designed so that information gathered at one time can be meaningfully compared with data obtained later; and they can be used to gather the relevant information at minimal cost of staff time. Several questionnaires are available for pain assessment. Many of these have been designed to be used with patients who have nonmalignant pain, or are too lengthy for repeated use or with very ill patients. Although it must be brief, the questionnaire must give a reasonable estimate of the patient's pain severity and its variability, as well as give a picture of the degree to which pain interferes with the patient's mood and functioning, thereby portraying the multidimensional aspects of the problem.

We have developed a questionnaire for assessing pain and its impact specifically for the cancer patient which we feel meets most of these goals [17]. This questionnaire, which is now called the Brief Pain Inventory, attempts to survey both the patient's pain severity as well as other aspects of the patient's functioning that may be affected by pain. The questionnaire asks patients whether or not they have had pain due to their illness in the last week. Those who are free of pain go to the end of the questionnaire to answer a brief survey of mood states, modified from the Profile of Mood States [18]. This helps identify patients who, although they do not have pain, do have a disturbance in mood that needs attention. Those who have pain also complete the mood questions, but also answer several questions describing their pain and its impact on them.

Using numeric scales, we ask the patients to rate, for the preceding week, the intensity of their pain at its maximum, minimum, and average severity. We also ask patients to rate their pain at the time the questionnaire is given. Patients are asked to rate the degree to which pain, in their perception, has interfered with several life

Table 3-1. Functions reported as impaired by cancer patients with different levels of pain severity

Function	Level of Pain Severity (0–10 Scales)
Enjoyment of life	3
Work	4
Sleep	5
Mood state	5
General activity	5
Walking	7
Relations with others	8

Function impairment = Interference rating of 4 or more (0–10 scales) for each function domain.

areas, including activity, mood, sleep, work, relationships with others, and capacity to enjoy life.

We also ask patients how much relief they get from treatment for pain and how long the relief lasts. We ask them which treatment for pain provides the best relief. We ask them to indicate, on a human figure drawing, the location of their pain. We finally ask them to rate various descriptors of the quality of their pain.

We have studied several issues of reliability and validity related to the questionnaire. To summarize these studies, satisfactory reliability exists for questions assessing pain and interference. Concurrent validity is suggested by the association of pain severity with expected correlates, such as disease extent and severity. Comparable information is obtained by self-administration and interviewer administration [17].

FACTORS RELATED TO PAIN SEVERITY

Standard assessment of the multidimensional aspects of cancer pain makes it clear that pain severity is the primary factor in determining the impact of pain on the patient. It is more important to know the severity of the pain than to know that the patient does or does not have pain. Many adults, both with and without cancer, function quite effectively with a background level of pain that, for the most part, does not seriously impair or distract them. As pain severity increases, however, it passes a threshold beyond which it cannot be ignored. At this point, it becomes disruptive to many aspects of the patient's life. At very high levels, pain becomes a primary focus of attention and prohibits most non-pain-related activity. Table 3-1 presents data indicating the relationship between increasing pain severity and the dimensions of life activity with which pain interferes.

PSYCHIATRIC AND BEHAVIORAL TREATMENT INDICATIONS

The minority of cancer patients who have psychiatric disease in addition to significant pain will need management of their psychiatric condition as a comorbidity of their cancer, just as the cancer patient with diabetes or heart disease will need to have attention paid to these elements of his or her medical condition. For the patient in pain, special concern will need to be given to the combined management of psychotropic medications and analgesics. In most cases, however, we should not assume that psychiatrically disturbed patients will require special consideration in judging their reports of pain severity or response to appropriate analgesic therapy.

One exception to this rule should be made for patients who have a history of a behavioral disorder in which complaints of having pain played a prominent role. Such patients may need special training to help them distinguish new complaints of pain from their chronic background level of discomfort. These patients need to be able to sort out new from old pain complaints so that it is possible to monitor pain as a sign of progressing disease and to prescribe an effective analgesic program.

All patients with active cancer need to be assertive in reporting pain when it is present, and in insisting that staff make every effort for its relief. Some patients will need special coaching to accomplish this. For these patients, this type of behavioral training may be the single most effective psychological strategy in helping them attain pain relief. In addition, all patients need information about the degree to which they can expect pain relief and how they can best comply with an analgesic program.

BEHAVIORAL PAIN-CONTROL METHODS

There is increasing evidence suggesting that it is possible to teach patients various psychological or self-control techniques that they can use to reduce the pain and discomfort associated with disease. Several names have been given to these methods, including cognitive behavior modification, behavioral skills training, and behavioral control techniques. For the purposes of this chapter, the term *behavioral control* will be used to mean all learned self-control measures, even though they are somewhat different from one another. These behavioral control techniques include hypnosis, autogenic training, cognitive control, methods of relaxation training, and training in physiological control using biofeedback. The common element among them is that they teach the patient specific skills that can be used in the control of discomfort. All of these techniques represent skills in the true sense of the word in that they require learning and practice before they can be applied. Patients do not acquire them passively; they have to be actively engaged in their acquisition and use. As with other skills, patients may develop increasing confidence in their ability to use them over time.

It is important to note that the effectiveness of behavioral control methods for cancer pain management has not been examined systematically. Most of the studies that do exist report outcome data on very small numbers of patients. At the same time, there is substantial evidence indicating that these techniques are effective with patients who have pain due to nonmalignant causes. Many of these nonmalignant conditions produce pain by very similar physiological mechanisms to those causing cancer pain, and in many instances the pain is of a similar severity.

Behavioral control techniques have many potential advantages for working with cancer pain. For the appropriate patient, the pain control achieved by the use of these techniques is essentially free of undesirable side effects. Cancer patients often complain of the lack of control they experience as a result of the demanding medical treatment that their cancer necessitates. Learning self-control measures may restore some sense of their own potency in dealing with their symptoms. In addition, these techniques can often be used to control other aspects of discomfort associated with the disease, including difficulty in sleeping, anticipatory nausea and vomiting, and anxiety associated with many of the procedures cancer patients must undergo.

One reason that these techniques have found limited application to the cancer patient is that their use has been seen as most appropriate for patients with emotional disturbance. Despite this prevailing assumption, patients who show the greatest potential for their use are those who do not have a major psychiatric disturbance. The patient with a psychiatric disorder may have difficulty in learning and recalling behavioral skills, or may not be motivated to use them. The normal distress that is present as a result of having cancer and of having pain often functions to motivate nondisturbed patients to learn these measures. Before introducing behavioral control to the patient, it is important to point out that using these techniques does not imply that the pain is psychogenic. Patients need to be reassured that no one is denying they have real pain. They also need to be reassured that no one intends to take away needed analgesics, even if they achieve some success in pain reduction using behavioral control.

INDICATIONS FOR VARIOUS BEHAVIORAL CONTROL THERAPIES

Behavioral control techniques have several common dimensions or elements, although each separate technique may emphasize one element over others. Three dimensions are probably most responsible for pain reduction: relaxation, distraction or redirection of attention, and an increased sense of self-control. These dimensions may be effective at the level of pain sensation, at the level of reaction to pain (sometimes called the affective component of pain), or at a combination of both levels at the same time.

Relaxation skills can reduce both the sensory as well as the reactive components of pain. At the level of pain sensation, muscle contraction may aggravate the sensitivity of tissue already compressed by tumor. Sympathetic overactivity may contribute to painful ischemia. Relaxation can directly influence pain sensation by reducing tonic muscle contraction or by increasing blood flow as a result of decreased sympathetic tone. Relaxation skills can also play a role in reducing the reactive component of pain by helping to control the anxiety associated with painful episodes and the increased vigilance associated with sustained pain.

. The mechanisms by which redirection of attention (or distraction) operate to reduce pain are not well understood. Some evidence suggests that redirection of attention may have some effect on pain transmission systems, thus affecting pain at the level of sensation. It is probable that redirection of attention also operates at the level of reaction to pain. There is sufficient laboratory evidence that distraction can reduce pain report, and patients often relate that distraction can have marked positive effects on how much pain they experience.

The third critical element in the pain-reducing effectiveness of behavioral control measures is the sense of increasing self-control that their use can impart. The cancer patient faces exacting schedules of anticancer therapies for a disease that often has an unpredictable course, reducing the patient's control over the conduct of his or her life. The presence of pain adds additional constraints to planning accomplishments. When patients develop a sense of having some mastery over the pain that they experience, a measure of self-efficacy is restored. This can serve to reduce anxiety and brighten mood, attenuating the reactive component of pain.

In deciding when behavioral control techniques will be of use for the individual patient, several aspects of the pain assessment should be considered. First, the severity of the pain should be taken into account. Patients with very mild pain that is easily controlled by nonnarcotic analgesics may not be good candidates for these measures, because they have little incentive to expend the time and effort required for learning them. Probably the best candidates for behavioral control are those who have pain of moderate severity that is only partially controlled by analgesics. Patients with severe pain *may* be candidates for distraction and redirection of attention, perhaps through hypnosis. Most of this last group, however, will probably have difficulty deriving benefits from more traditional relaxation techniques. It is important to remember that pain severity will change due to both the progression of the disease as well as its treatment. For example, some patients with severe pain may, later in their disease, have moderate pain for which behavioral methods are indicated. Pain may be reduced by response to anticancer therapy or more effective analgesic management. The assessment should also consider the temporal pattern of the pain. Pain that is relatively constant may dictate a behavioral measure such as relaxation, whereas distraction or another cognitive control method may be most useful for pain that is episodic in nature.

Preparation for the use of behavioral control techniques should also include a careful assessment of the cognitive and behavioral dimensions of the patient's response to pain. Patients may misperceive the nature of the pain itself or their ability to cope with it. Clarification of these misperceptions may be especially helpful in reducing pain-related distress. For example, a patient's impression that pain is inevitable needs to be corrected. Patients may respond to periods of pain with self-statements that amplify their reaction to the pain or may even augment the transmission of pain sensation. Such statements may include thoughts about inability to cope with pain, the horrible nature of the pain that they are experiencing, or the lack of the ability of family and staff to help reduce the pain. Occasionally, some patients may misperceive non-malignant pain as cancer related. A review of the pain-related self-statements during the assessment can be therapeutic in itself when misperceptions can be corrected and realistic goals established.

The selection of a behavioral control technique can be assisted by a knowledge of the physical basis of the pain. Studies of patients with moderately severe to severe cancer pain have shown that about 50% have pain due to tumor infiltration of bone. An additional 25% have pain due to involvement of nerve, with the remainder having pain due either to the involvement of soft tissue or to posttherapy complications. Patients with pain due to nerve or soft-tissue involvement may respond especially well to appropriate relaxation techniques. Posttherapy pain, such as that produced by radiation fibrosis, is also a target for relaxation approaches. This later type of pain has much in common with chronic myofascial pain, a condition where relaxation techniques have been shown to be a benefit. Pain due to infiltration of bone is the most resistant to the effects of any pain therapy, and the same difficulty can be anticipated for behavioral control techniques. If secondary muscle spasm is present, relaxation techniques may help control that component of pain. Redirection of attention may provide for periods of escape from pain. Finally, behavioral control may help the patient with bone pain modify his or her reaction to the pain.

TECHNIQUES OF BEHAVIORAL CONTROL

Because it shares elements with many other behavioral control techniques, biofeedback training is a good place to start our review of specific behavioral control measures. Biofeedback involves the use of electronic physiological monitoring equipment for the purpose of facilitating the learning of control over physiological responses. Learning to improve our performance of any skill without information about how we are progressing is extremely difficult. When that information is not available to us, learning may be impossible. This is the case with many physiological functions. Detectors and amplifiers are now available which can provide information about muscle activity, blood pressure, skin temperature, brain activity, and blood flow. When we have immediate access to these events, it is sometimes possible to modify them. Muscle or EMG biofeedback is very helpful in teaching relaxation. We normally get some information from our muscles without external feedback, but usually only when they are very tight, sometimes as pain. Biofeedback helps the patient detect very small changes in muscle contraction, leading the way to a more relaxed state in small steps. Biofeedback allows the patient to detect these small steps and learn what produces them.

Other types of relaxation training must also proceed gradually. It is difficult to move rapidly from a state of chronic muscle contraction to deep relaxation. Progressive relaxation training, sometimes abbreviated PRT, is a nonbiofeedback method of producing deep muscle relaxation. This method is summarized by Bernstein and Borkovec [19]. Here, the patient learns to sense muscle tension by contracting, then relaxing, several different muscle groups of the body. Each muscle group is dealt with in a systematic order that can be repeated from session to session.

There is another set of skills that patients can learn that are especially useful in dealing with sympathetic overarousal. In the biofeedback arena, skin–temperature control is useful for this purpose. Here, a small thermistor (or electronic thermometer) is attached to the skin, usually to the fingers or toes. Patients are coached to gradually increase the temperature of this body part. Increasing skin temperature reflects increased blood flow to the body part. As we relax sympathetically, peripheral blood flow is increased, and increasing skin temperature can be used as an index of reduced sympathetic arousal. There are also nonbiofeedback ways of producing these changes. One is autogenic training. The patients are given a set of self-statements dealing with warmth, heaviness, and calm to say to themselves several times over. Despite the simplicity of this technique, its ability to produce deep relaxation is very powerful. A related behavioral method is training in rhythmic breathing. Here, the patient is encouraged to breathe slowly, deeply, and smoothly. This technique has parallels with yoga and other nonwestern forms of deep relaxation.

Hypnosis is the best example of a powerful distraction technique. Whatever else happens in hypnosis, the attention of the person is dramatically focused on the suggestions being offered and the images being created. The hypnotic induction is designed to focus attention. It defines the time devoted to hypnosis as a very special time. Hypnosis can also produce profound relaxation. The mystique of hypnosis amplifies its usefulness. Most of the general public think of hypnosis as a very powerful technique. This is often helpful for cancer patients, some of whom think that only a very powerful measure will be of help for their pain. Those who plan to use hypnosis should plan to dedicate considerable time to learning the technique before applying it. There is some risk in using the technique. Patients may experience a release of emotional feelings during hypnosis and the practitioner needs to be prepared to guide the patient through this release.

Certain cognitive control techniques parallel hypnotic suggestions, but do not use the hypnotic induction [20]. It is possible that these techniques may be as effective (or nearly as effective) as the same material presented following hypnotic induction. Since no hypnotic induction is required, these measures can be used by larger numbers of health care staff. They include such manipulations as sensory transformation of the pain, where the patient is encouraged to relabel the sensations from the painful area; for example, "painful" sensations may also be relabeled as "pressure" or "numb." Some of these techniques are entirely directed at helping the patient restructure how they react to pain. For example, patients are encouraged to reinforce themselves for coping well despite pain. Patients are also encouraged to prepare for predictable periods of episodic pain, and not to rehearse these episodes in their minds once they have passed.

In the initial presentation of behavioral control methods to cancer patients, it is important to acknowledge that these skills will not control all of the pain all of the time. A sense of failure is the most serious potential negative side effect of behavioral control training. The patient should be encouraged to take an experimental attitude, presented as "Let's see how well some of these methods might work to reduce some of your pain." Since the severity, source, and temporal pattern of pain in cancer may differ from time to time, it is helpful to teach several pain control techniques to each patient. This serves to reinforce an experimental attitude as well as the expectation that no one skill will be equally effective in all painful situations.

APPLICATIONS WITH DIFFERENT PATIENT GROUPS

At different stages in their disease, patients will experience unique problems with pain in terms of its severity, impact on activities, and meaning to the patient. The special features of pain at these different stages calls for specifically tailored behavioral control training. Four groups of patients present the most common pain control problems that will be faced [21].

The patient preparing for intensive anticancer therapy that will produce pain

Most treatment-related pain, including postsurgical pain, can be managed adequately using analgesics. With the development of newer, more heroic treatment methods (including extensive surgery, bone-marrow transplantation, and hyperthermia), some patients will experience severe, time-limited pain related to their therapy. These patients need to be made aware of their need to report pain during therapy and to insist on adequate pain management. Patients need information upon which to base their evaluation of analgesic effectiveness. It is useful to inform them about the expected duration of analgesia from the medications that they are taking, the need to maintain a blood level of analgesic sufficient to protect them from pain, and the negligible risk of psychological addiction should opiate drugs be required for a specific time during their treatment.

Patients facing a planned period of painful therapy may also benefit from specific behavioral control training if sufficient time for training exists before therapy begins. Training in relaxation, with or without the aid of biofeedback, can give the patient specific skills in managing the reactive components of pain during the period of therapy. Training in self-hypnosis can give patients a powerful distraction technique, especially useful for treatment-related pain that is episodic in nature. It may be especially useful for the patient to develop, through self-hypnosis, a vivid image of a specific comfortable place, created with the help of fantasy or recall. Patients can then envisage themselves in this comfortable place when therapy becomes distressing. Both relaxation and self-hypnosis instructions can be tape-recorded, which allows the patient to review them during the anticancer therapy.

The patient with active disease with a prognosis of several months

Patients with pain who have an indefinite prognosis are often excellent candidates for effective use of behavioral control methods. While many of them will be maintained on analgesics, including opiates, they may wish to limit their use of these drugs to avoid negative side effects, especially mental blurring. Many will wish to continue working, to engage fully in family activities, and to pursue meaningful avocational interests. Some patients may want to learn these measures to control other areas of distress associated with their disease and its treatment, including anticipatory reactions to therapy, generalized anxiety, and difficulty in going to sleep.

The behavioral control techniques having the greatest potential application to this group of patients are quite similar to those useful for the previous group, although the scope of these potential use is greater. These patients will have a continuing need for pain control skills, not limited to the duration of a sepecific therapy. They will also have more time for the training and refinement of skills. Those providing behavior training should assure themselves that the patient has a reasonable knowledge of the place of analgesics in their pain management, along the lines of the information provided to the group undergoing painful treatment. These patients, however, will need a greater painful treatment. These patients, however, will need a greater appreciation for the need to take analgesics on a continuing basis, including how to minimize the chronic negative side effects of these medications.

The specific technique to be selected should be based on careful assessment of the pain, including its physical basis, location, temporal pattern, and the pattern of interference with activity that it causes for the individual patient. Training in muscle relaxation will be of benefit for patients with a muscle spasm component to their pain, or for whom pain is exacerbated by muscle traction on pain-sensitive areas. Relaxation training can also be useful for reducing pain-produced anxiety and for helping the patient get to sleep despite the presence of pain. When pain is produced by reduced blood flow, training in skin-temperature warming, with its associated increase in blood flow, may provide pain relief. This type of training can be achieved with skin-temperature biofeedback or with autogenic suggestions.

Training in self-hypnosis is often useful for this group. As with the patient undergoing painful anticancer therapy, self-hypnosis can be used for the development of an image of a pleasant location that can provide a respite from pain and other disease-associated distress. Self-hypnosis can also be used to aid the patient in attempts to transform the sensation of the pain into a less noxious one, for instance, from "painful" to "numb." Similar cognitive manipulations can also be done without hypnotic induction.

Exploration of the thoughts and feelings provoked by the pain can be helpful. Some patients may set unrealistically high goals for themselves in spite of their pain and other limitations imposed by their disease. Others may not appropriately reinforce themselves for being active in the face of pain. By contrast, some patients will unnecessarily limit their activity and augment their pain by rehearsing thoughts about how horrible their pain is and how hopeless they are to cope with it.

The patient in the terminal stages of illness

Cancer patients are at greatest risk for severe pain at the end of their life. The majority of patients with solid tumors will suffer significant pain during this time. This period calls for careful medical pain management, including evaluation for surgical or anesthetic ablation of pain pathways. Often, the patient's role in reporting both pain and lack of adequate pain control will have to be assumed by family members. The role of behavioral control procedures is less clear at this point. Patients have little time to devote to learning and practicing new skills, and their time is rightfully focused on family.

Some patients may request hypnosis to help them cope with pain during end-stage disease. Hypnotic induction, however, can be compromised by the severity of pain, the presence of brain metastases, and the obtunding effects of opiate analgesics and other drugs. Rather than teach self-hypnosis, an option is to offer direct suggestions for comfort and deep relaxations. The hypnotic induction, coupled with appropriate suggestions, can be recorded on tape so that the patient can use it when desired.

The patient with no active disease but with persistent post-treatment pain

Some patients who, by all available evidence, are cured of their cancer will have persistent chronic pain due to the treatments that they have undergone. This pain can be produced by postsurgical scarring, neuropathy induced by chemo- or radio-therapy, or postirradiation myelopathy or fibrosis. Those who undergo amputation for osteosarcoma are at risk for persistent phantom-limb pain. The most common basis for most of these pain syndromes is treatment-related destruction of nerve. This often causes a burning pain and dyesthesias which are extremely unpleasant but difficult for patients to describe. The pain may have its onset weeks or months after the termination of treatment. In contrast to the other three groups of patients previously discussed, it is generally agreed that patients in this group are not candidates for continued opiate analgesic therapy. The behavioral management approach to these patients is quite similar to that for patients who endure chronic pain due to nonmalignant causes.

As with other patients with chronic pain, relaxation training can be of major benefit to these patients. Frequently, sustained muscle contraction or even muscle spasm may occur in reaction to the primary pain and significantly augment the total pain the patient experiences. Training can use either EMG biofeedback or progressive muscle relaxation.

When treatment-induced nerve damage causes pain via the mechanism of decreased blood flow, training in skin-temperature increases might be tried either via biofeedback or autogenic suggestion. This training has most frequently found application for the ischemia-induced symptoms of Raynaud's phenomenon and disease. The technique has also been applied to patients with frequent migraine headache. No controlled studies of its application to the specific pain syndromes induced by autonomic nerve damage have been reported, although several case studies have been offered in support of this application.

As with patients having chronic pain due to noncancer causes, physiological training for symptom reduction is probably rarely effective in isolation. Persons with chronic pain are at risk for a number of negative behavioral consequences of their condition. They may need a variety of cognitive control strategies to help them cope with their pain. They may need to reorganize self-statements that exaggerate the negative consequences of having pain, and most will need to learn to positively reinforce themselves for increased activity. During the assessment procedure, it should be determined whether or not the patient has developed specific problems as a cancer survivor. During the time when they had active disease, a minority of patients may have received increased attention and support from both family and friends that was not present before they had a life-threatening illness. Such patients are at risk for focusing on pain as a way of maintaining the support they previously had. For these patients, a reappraisal of their current situation, coupled with learning skills that allow them to obtain social reinforcement in more adaptive ways, may reduce their need to focus on their pain. When this fails, patients might wish to consider participating in a highly structured inpatient or outpatient pain management program, designed to reinforce increased activity and reorganize the consequences of being in pain.

CONCLUSIONS

Pain of increasing severity inevitably has negative consequences for the psychological well-being of the cancer patient. As pain becomes more severe, it increasingly intrudes on the patient's mood and activity and becomes a preoccupying concern. When pain severity is reduced through adequate pain management, its intrusiveness is reversed. Patients newly diagnosed with cancer will expect their disease to be painful, their treatment for cancer to add to their pain, and will worry that potent analgesics needed to control severe pain will put them at risk for addiction and intolerable negative side effects. Despite the adverse effect of pain on mood, the evidence suggests that depression does not contribute to the reporting of pain as more severe, nor does it necessarily stand in the way of a good response to adequate pain management. Patients with preexisting psychiatric disease need parallel management for both their psychiatric problems and their pain.

For all patients with cancer-related pain, behavioral techniques can play a role in comprehensive pain management. At the most elementary level, patients with active disease need to be taught to report their pain and to communicate to staff when pain-relief measures are not working. Systematic assessment of pain and its consequences facilitate patient–staff communication about pain.

At a second level, patients can learn specific skills to help them manage their pain and its impact on their lives. A wide variety of such skills are available that can be tailored to the individual patient's needs and the stage of disease where pain presents a problem. For the disease-free patient who has persistent treatment-related pain, behavioral techniques may represent the treatment of choice. When active disease is present, however, behavioral techniques will always be adjunctive to appropriate analgesic management.

REFERENCES

1. Cleeland CS (1984): Impact of pain on the patient with cancer. Cancer 54:2635.
2. Levin CN, Cleeland CS, Dar R (1985): Public attitudes towards cancer pain. Cancer 56(9): 2337–2339.
3. Ahles TA, Blanchard EB, Ruchdeschel JC (1983): Multidimensional nature of cancer pain. Pain 17:277–288.
4. McKegney FP, Bailey LR, Yates JW (1981): Prediction and management of pain in patients with advanced cancer. Gen Hosp Psychiat 3:95–101.
5. Bond MR (1979): Psychologic and emotional aspects of cancer pain. In: Bonica JJ, Ventafridda V (eds), Advances in Pain Research and Therapy, vol 2. New York: Raven Press, 81–88.
6. Spiegel D, Bloom JR (1983): Pain in metastatic breast cancer. Cancer 52:341–345.
7. Bukberg JB, Penman DT, Holland JC (1984): Depression in hospitalized cancer patients. Psychosomat Med 46:199–212.
8. Schwab JJ, Bialow M, Brown JM, et al. (1967): Diagnosing depression in medical inpatients. Ann Intern Med 67(4):695–707.
9. Moffic H, Paykel ES (1975): Depression in medical inpatients. Br J Psychiat 126:346–353.
10. Woodforde JM, Fielding JR (1975): Pain and cancer. In: Weisenburg M (ed), Pain, Clinical and Experimental Perspectives. St. Louis: C.V. Mosby, pp 332–336.

11. Shacham S, Reinhardt LC, Raubertas RF, Cleeland CS (1983): Emotional state and pain: Intraindividual and interindividual measures of association. J Behav Med 6:405–419.
12. Cleeland CS, Cleeland LM, Dar R, Reinhardt LC (1986): Factors influencing physician management of cancer pain. Cancer 58:796–800.
13. Marks RN, Sacher EJ (1973): Undertreatment of medical inpatients with narcotic analgesics. Ann Int Med 78:173.
14. Zborowski M (1969): People In Pain. San Francisco: Jojsey-Bass.
15. Harris IB, Rich EC, Crowson TW (1985): Attitudes of internal medicine residents and staff toward various patient characteristics. J Med Ed 60.
16. Cleeland CS (1985): Measurement & prevalence of pain in cancer 1983. Sem Nurs Onc 2:87–92.
17. Daut RL, Cleeland CS, Flanery RC (1983): Development of the Wisconsin brief pain questionnaire to assess pain in cancer and other diseases. Pain 17:197–210.
18. Shacham S (1983): A shortened version of the Profile of Mood States. J Pers Assess 47:305–306.
19. Bernstein DA, Borkovec TD (1973): Progressive relocation training: A manual for the helping professions. Champaign, IL: Research Press.
20. Turk D, Meichenbaum, Genest M (1983): Pain and behavioral medicine. New York: Guilford Press.
21. Cleeland CS, Tearnan BH (1986): Behavioral control of cancer pain. In: Hozman AD, Turk DC (eds), Pain Management. New York: Pergamon.

4. RADIOTHERAPY, CHEMOTHERAPY AND HORMONAL THERAPY IN THE MANAGEMENT OF CANCER PAIN: PUTTING PATIENT, PROGNOSIS, AND ONCOLOGIC OPTIONS IN PERSPECTIVE

ROSS A. ABRAMS, M.D.
RICHARD M. HANSEN, M.D.

When an oncologist encounters a patient with a suspected or histologically proven diagnosis of malignancy, he will, in the course of his clinical assessment, seek answers to the following questions.

1. What are the patient's symptoms; what is their degree of severity?

2. Are the patient's symptoms consistent with the remainder of the clinical findings, e.g., physical exam, laboratory tests, radiographic examinations? Are additional tests required?

3. Is the diagnosis of malignancy established histologically? If established, does the known clinical biology of the malignancy in question fit with the pattern of disease seen in this particular patient? Is it likely that there is some other, nonmalignant disease process causing the observed symptoms or findings?

4. What therapeutic options are available for managing the malignant disease in this patient? Have any of these options already been utilized? What effect did they have on the patient's situation?

5. How severely debilitated is the patient by his malignant disease; what is his performance status? Prognosis?

6. What therapeutic goals are reasonable—cure, some interval of disease-free survival, attempt at partial response? Should there be no attempt at controlling the underlying malignancy? Should therapeutic efforts be focused mainly on symptom control rather than disease control?

7. What are the negative consequences and toxicities of the various therapeutic choices under consideration? Do they seem reasonable when compared to the desired therapeutic goal and the estimated probability of reaching this desired goal? If the balance between toxicity and benefit seems appropriate to the involved physicians, is there concurrence with this assessment on the part of the patient and family?

8. If a major effort is to be made at controlling the patient's malignant process through the use of various antineoplastic modalities (e.g., surgery, radiation, chemotherapy, or their combination), what methods of symptom control need be implemented on an interim basis?

The scope of this chapter precludes a full discussion of each of these issues. However, by allowing ourselves to focus primarily on issues related to the management of cancer *pain*, we must not allow ourselves to overlook the inherently important questions raised above as they relate to the overall issues of optimizing management of the patient's *cancer*.

The term *cancer pain* might well bring to mind an image of a prior patient or relative stricken with metastatic cancer, in bed, debilitated, cachectic, preterminal with severe pain from bone destruction or obstructed viscus. Although such circumstances regretfully do occur, we must bear in mind that there is far more to cancer management (and the management of cancer pain) than providing care for patients whose circumstances fit this unfortunate stereotypical image. In one sense, the best control of cancer pain is to control the cancer and thereby prevent, or at least delay, its symptomatic manifestations, including pain.

Cancer per se is a process, not a diagnosis. A specific diagnosis related to cancer usually requires identification of an organ of origin as well as specific histology, e.g., small-cell carcinoma of the lung, transitional-cell carcinoma of the bladder, adenocarcinoma of the breast. Once identified, the malignancy is usually staged. Staging systems vary by organ site but typically include assessment of the size and extent of the primary tumor, the presence, size, and extent of regional lymph node involvement, and the presence and extent of evidence to suggest hematogenous (distant, systemic) metastases. Insight into the overall impact of the malignant process can be further characterized by assessing degree of weight loss (if any) and by quantitating the patient's performance status, i.e., the ability of the patient to carry on the activities of daily living (table 4-1).

With this information in hand, the informed oncologist, aware of probabilities for effecting cure, interval control, or palliation (table 4-2) with available antineoplastic therapies, can formulate an approporiate therapeutic strategy based either on disease control, symptom control, or their combination in some degree. Certainly, such an analysis should be carefully undertaken before patients are approached primarily with palliative intent.

With these general considerations in mind, we may more properly turn our attention to the use of radiotherapy, chemotherapy, and hormonal therapy for controlling pain in patients with incurable malignancy.

Table 4-1. Performance Status Assessment

Karnofsky Scale	ECOG* (Zubrod) Scale
100 Normal; no complaints, no disease	0 — Asymptomatic
90 Normal activity level; minimal signs or symptoms of disease	1 — Symptomatic, Ambulatory
80 Normal activity with effort, some signs or symptoms of disease	

70 Unable to work or do normal activity
  Able to do self care
	2 — Symptomatic.
	  In bed <50% of day

60 Able to do most self care	
50 Needs considerable assistance for self care and frequent medical care	3 — Symptomatic. In bed >50% of day
40 Disabled	
30 Severely disabled	4 — Bedridden
20 Very sick; hospitalization required	
10 Moribund	
00 Dead	

* ECOG — Eastern Co-operative Oncologic Group.

RADIATION THERAPY

Radiation therapy refers to the use of any of several types of irradiations to control or palliate human disease, usually some form of malignant disease. The physics and specific biological considerations that are germane to the proper utilization of irradiation are, in general, not always well understood by those who are not radiation therapists This, in turn, may lead to some misconceptions regarding the proper role and consequences of management with this modality. Consequently, brief review of some basic principles seems in order.

Radiation therapy can be administered in one of two ways: by utilization of a beam of irradiation from a properly collimated, quantitated, and directed external source, as is commonly done with Cobalt-60 or linear accelerator therapy units, or by the direct juxtaposition of a radionuclide of desired activity and geometry next to or within body tissues or cavities. Therapy delivered from external sources at distance is usually referred to as teletherapy; therapy delivered by the juxtaposition or insertion of radionuclides close to or within the body is referred to as brachytherapy. Both forms of therapy may have definite application for purposes of palliation, although teletherapy is the more frequently utilized modality with respect to pain control. The interested reader will find additional sources of information regarding brachytherapy in the bibliography. The remainder of this discussion will focus on pain palliation with teletherapy.

In designing a treatment plan incorporating the palliative use of external beam radiation therapy, the managing physician needs to define a target volume containing the locus of symptomatic tumor with some margin of normal tissue. This target volume must then be related in three dimensions to the patient's surrounding

Table 4-2A. Examples of possible curative results by site, histology, and stage: Initial treatment—adult malignancies

Organ	Disease	Stage	Therapeutic Goal	Treatment
Brain	Grade I/II glioma	N/A	Cure, long-term disease-free survival	Surgery, surgery and irradiation
Upper aerodigestive tract	Typically squamous cell cancer	I–III	Cure, long-term disease-free survival	Surgery, irradiation, surgery and irradiation
		IV	Rare to occasional cure, prevent local recurrence/progression	Surgery, irradiation, surgery and irradiation
Lung	Small cell	Limited	Cure (10–20%), temporary disease control	Chemotherapy irradiation
Lung	Non-small cell	I, II, III	Cure or locoregional control	Surgery, surgery and irradiation, irradiation
Colorectal	Adenocarcinoma	Dukes A, B, C	Cure, prevention of local recurrence	Surgery Surgery and irradiation
Sarcoma	Varied	I–III	Cure, preservation of functional extremity, prevent local recurrence	Surgery and irradiation ± chemotherapy
Lymphoma	Diffuse	I	Cure	Irradiation
		II	Cure	Chemotherapy and irradiation
		III, IV	Cure	Chemotherapy, irradiation or their combination
	Hodgkins	I–IV	Cure	Chemotherapy, irradiation, or chemotherapy and irradiation
Breast	Adenocarcinoma	I–III	Cure, disease control	Surgery, irradiation, adjuvant chemotherapy
Cervix	Squamous	I–III	Cure, local control	Surgery, irradiation, or their combination

anatomy, taking into account the specific biologic response of surrounding normal tissues to irradiation, the time course over which these responses may be expected, and any past history of prior irradiation to these tissues.

Modern radiation therapy has been greatly facilitated by the availability of megavoltage-range linear accelerators capable of producing very high-energy x-rays or electron beams. Simplistically stated, linear accelerators are capable of raising the

Table 4–2B. Examples of options available for
management of disseminated disease: adult malignancy

1. Chemotherapy with curative intent	Hodgkin's lymphoma, non-Hodgkins lymphoma, testicular carcinoma, choriocarcinoma, acute leukemia
2. Symptomatic relief	Painful or symptomatic metastases to bone, brain, liver; management with irradiation (see text) or chemotherapy (see text)
3. Short-term disease control with chemotherapy clearly helpful	Disseminated breast, small-cell lung cancer (extensive), ovarian cancer (stage III, IV)
4. Tumors responsive to hormonal manipulations	Breast, endometrial, prostate

Table 4–3[a]. Depth of maximal dose by x-ray beam energy (5 cm × 5 cm field)

Type of X-Ray Beam	Depth of Maximal Dose
Orthovoltage	Surface
Cobalt-60	0.5 cm
6 MV linear accelerator	1.5 cm
10 MV linear accelerator	2.5 cm
25 MV linear accelerator	4.0 cm

[a] Modified from Johns HE, Cunningham JR (1983): The Physics of Radiology, 4th ed. Springfield: C.C. Thomas, Appendix B.

potential energy of electrons by millions of volts (megavolts). These electrons may then be either used to treat the patient directly or directed at a target within the linear accelerator itself to produce x-rays of megavoltage levels of energy to treat the patient. Megavoltage x-rays have as a primary advantage the sparing of superficial tissues (table 4–3). In other words, as a beam of megavoltage x-rays penetrates the patient, the majority of energy carried by the x-rays is transferred to the patient's tissues at some depth under the skin. By combining this fortuitous property with the use of multiple fields aimed at the target volume from different angles or direction, very significant doses of irradiation can be administered to deeply situated tumor masses with significant sparing of skin and other superficial tissues. Consequently, the undesired severe, acute radiation reactions of skin and subcutaneous tissues seen previously in association with less powerful x-ray machines (kilovoltage range) should now largely be a thing of the past in the treatment of deeply seated, visceral deposits of metastatic malignancy.

In defining a treatment prescription, the radiation therapist has multiple parameters to specify in addition to the target volume, choice of fields, and nature and energy of irradiation to be utilized. Such choices include dose per treatment, frequency of treatments, and total dose to be administered. Each of these parameters can in turn have profound impact on the biologic result produced both in tumor and normal tissue. Moreover, there is no easy formula that will accurately translate a set of parameters to a common biologic effect with respect to tumor response, acute normal tissue effects, and late normal tissue effects. Thus, comparison of one radiotherapeutic treatment regimen with other possible radiotherapeutic treatment regimens is difficult in spite of efforts that have been made in this direction [1,2]. In the final analysis, such comparisons can be based most reliably only on clinical experience.

Ideally, radiotherapy treatment plans administered with palliative intent would be given with relatively few fractions in order to minimize the burden of the treatment experience. Unfortunately, increased fraction size runs the risk of increasing late damage to normal tissues, especially potentially irreversibly sensitive structures such as spinal cord and brain [3]. Additionally, there may be risk that such hypofractionated treatment regimens may be less effective at producing tumor control and palliation. Several studies (discussed below) have attempted to examine these issues.

Sites where radiation therapy may be helpful in pain control (table 4.2B)

As reviewed by Bosch [4] and by Rechter and Coia [5], radiation therapy can be used palliatively to control pain, relieve obstruction, and decrease bleeding. Painful manifestations that may often be well relieved by irradiation include discomfort due to bone metastases and/or epidural cord or nerve root compression, headache due to brain metastases or primary brain malignancies, pain related to massive hepatic metastases, and deep pain related to advanced local progression of gynecologic, gastro-intestinal, or upper aerodigestive tract malignancies.

Management of bone pain with irradiation

Almost any disseminated malignancy can, in its final stages, be associated with bony metastases. However, in published series, the most frequently noted primary sites of malignancy among patients with symptomatic bony metastases are prostate, breast, and lung, a pattern reflecting both the frequency of these common malignancies and their propensity for dissemination to bone. Other noteworthy primary malignancies that may disseminate in bone include myeloma, lymphoma, thyroid carcinoma, melanoma, bladder, kidney, and occasionally malignancies originating in the gastrointestinal (colo-rectal, gastric, pancreatic) or gynecologic (endometrial, cervical) tracts.

Bony metastases are most commonly multiple rather than single and more frequently occur in the bones of the axial skeleton or proximal long bones [6]. Metastases in weight-bearing bones (spine, pelvis, femur) may jeopardize bony integrity with risk of pathologic fracture. In the presence of pathologic fracture or in the presence of significant cortical destruction without fracture (more than 30% loss of cortex on plain radio-graph), successful management usually involves therapeutic or prophylactic orthopedic intervention (pinning), respectively, in addition to irradiation to preserve function and obtain optimal pain control [6].

Pain is a *subjective* manifestation of disease, and therefore difficult to measure in objective terms. In 1976, Hendrickson et al. [7] published a scale for grading pain from zero to nine based on the presence or absence of pain, its frequency, duration, requirement for analgesics, and the type of analgesic required (nonnarcotic, narcotic). Later, Tong et al. [8], reporting Radiation Therapy Oncology Group (RTOG) results, refined this approach further. They scored each of the following parameters on a scale from zero to three: pain severity, pain frequency (by site), type of analgesic, frequency of analgesic. Changes in pain score (pain severity score × pain frequency score) and narcotic score (analgesic type score × analgesic frequency score) were then used to describe treatment results.

Using this methodologic approach for scoring response, Hendrickson et al. [7] reported that

1) Within two weeks of completing a course of radiotherapy, 54% of patients with prostate cancer, 79% of patients with lung cancer, and 80% of patients with breast cancer had improved their pain score by at least two levels;

2) By 13 weeks these percentages had changed to 80%, 79% (no change), and 72%, respectively; and

3) There was no apparent difference in efficacy of less intensive regimens (900 cGy* × 1 treatment, 600 cGy × 2 treatments, 300 cGy × 5 treatments, 200 cGy × 10 treatments) versus more intensive regimens (400 cGy × 5 treatments, 300 cGy × 10 treatments).

In a similar study, Allen et al. [9] reported that 70% of 152 patients experienced pain relief within two weeks of completing radiation therapy, and that 91% achieved pain relief within two months. As before [7], the *biologic* intensity of the treatment regimen as judged by nominal standard dose [9] did not predict for either probability of achieving pain relief or probability of failure after pain relief.

Tong et al. [8] reported the results of the RTOG following the completion of a prospectively conducted study that randomized patients with a single site of osseous metastases to receive 4050 cGy in three weeks versus 2000 cGy in one week, and patients with multiple metastases to receive 3000 cGy in two weeks or any one of the following in one week—1500 cGy, 2000 cGy, 2500 cGy. A total of 1016 patients were entered with 759 ultimately being evaluable. Within each patient group (solitary, multiple sites) there was no difference by treatment regimen with respect to frequency of pain relief or extent of pain relief. Overall, 54% of patients experienced complete pain relief and 83% partial pain relief. Median duration of complete pain relief was 15 weeks among patients with solitary sites of lung disease and 12 weeks among patients with multiple sites of bony disease. This study was subsequently reanalyzed by Blitzer [10]. He observed that when the results observed in the solitary site of disease group were pooled with the multiple site group, the regimens utilizing greater number of treatments per course (10 or 15) were more likely to result in complete relief as judged by both pain and narcotic scores than regimens utilizing fewer treatments per course.

---

* cGy = centigray; one centigray = 1 RAD. Formerly, the RAD was the accepted unit of absorbed radiation dose. The currently accepted dose unit is the gray. One gray is equivalent to one joule of absorbed energy per kilogram of tissue. One centigray is 0.01 gray.

For patients with very extensive bony metastases, a number of authors have reported the use of half-body irradiation—that is, the use of a single large field incorporating (usually) either the upper or lower body (including, as logically appropriate, head and upper extremities or lower extremities). Treatment is usually given as a single fraction in the range of 5–10 Gy (500–1000 cGy) with appropriate monitoring and management with respect to acute toxicity (nausea, vomiting, malaise, prostration) and acute toxicity (pulmonary, hematologic) [11–17].

Salazar et al. [12,17], reporting for the RTOG, found that approximately 67% of patients achieved clinically meaningful pain palliation (30% achieved complete pain relief) following half-body irradiation. Toxicity was significant but manageable. Severe acute toxicity was limited to patients receiving upper half-body irradiation and could be minimized by utilizing steroids, antiemetics, and intravenous hydration. Subacute pulmonary toxicity resulted in a 10–20% incidence of fatal pneumonitis when 800 cGy, single fraction, were given without correction for lung transmission, but this was not a problem at doses of 600 cGy. Hematologic toxicity was definite but not life-threatening, with recovery of counts in six to eight weeks.

Excellent results utilizing single doses of half-body irradiation were subsequently reported for patients with prostate cancer [13], multiple myeloma [14], and breast, prostate, and lung cancer [16,17]. Of particular interest is the consistent observation that many patients experienced pain relief within 24–48 *hours* of treatment.

Palliation of pain due to massive hepatic metastases

Multiple, massive hepatic metastases may be associated with a number of clinically distressing symptoms (nausea, anorexia, abdominal distention) including significant pain. When large portions of the liver (both lobes, multiple metastases) are involved, resection is generally not feasible, and many of the gastrointestinal and pulmonary epithileal neoplasms eventuating in hepatic metastases are only marginally or partially responsive to systemic chemotherapy. Fortunately, a number of studies [18–21] have clearly shown that anywhere from 55–90% of patients receiving external beam irradiation to the whole liver will experience durable relief of pain, lasting for approximately 60% to 80% of the remainder of the life of the patients so managed [20]. Additionally [20,21], hepatic irradiation is generally well tolerated and may also produce relief of the other symptoms associated with massive hepatic metastases, e.g., nausea, anorexia, distention.

Considering the relatively limited tolerance of the liver to irradiation, with acute radiation hepatitis becoming increasingly likely as doses in excess of 3000 cGy (conventional fractionation, 180–200 cGy per day, five days/week) are exceeded, the efficacy of external beam irradiation in producing pain relief is all the more noteworthy. Acute radiation hepatitis may occur within four to six weeks of completion of treatment and is generally characterized by hepatomegaly, striking elevations in serum levels of alkaline phosphatase, and histologic evidence of veno-occlusive changes involving the central hepatic veins [21]. Although in the absence of histologic examination of hepatic tissues such a syndrome might be difficult to distinguish from progression of metastatic disease, most workers have in fact concluded that within the dose limits described above, acute radiation effects have not been limiting. In fact, the RTOG examined a number of different fractionation schemes (e.g., 3000 cGy/15 fractions, 2500 cGy/16 fractions, 2000 cGy/10 fractions, 2100 cGy/7 fractions) in patients with multiple hepatic metastases, and found that none were associated with acute radiation hepatitis and all were seemingly effective (among relatively small patient groups) in producing pain relief (20).

The RTOG also observed that 1) pain relief was more frequent among patients with severe pain (70% relief) than among patients with mild pain (27% relief); 2) pain relief occurred in 64% of patients with serum bilirubin ≤1.5 mg% versus 38% with bilirubin >1.5 mg%; and 3) pain relief was somewhat more common among ambulatory than nonambulatory patients (67% versus 49%).

A number of studies have described the concomitant administration of chemotherapy, either systemic or via the hepatic artery, along with external irradiation [reviewed in 21]. When potentially confounding factors such as performance status, weight loss, pain treatment, and patient selection are borne in mind, it is difficult to know from available reports whether such combined modality efforts offer benefit over irradiation or chemotherapy alone.

Palliation of headache due to brain metastases

The management of intracerebral metastases with irradiation has been well described [22–28]. Early studies undertaken by the RTOG [26] and others [22] examined whether treatment courses of one or two relatively large fractions, e.g., 1500 cGy in two fractions or 1000 cGy in one fraction would be as effective as more conventional regimens of 2000, 3000, or 4000 cGy in two, three, or four weeks, respectively. The short course regimens (ultrarapid treatment regimens) were comparable in terms of percent of patients responding to the more conventional regimens [23–25], but also seemed to be associated with a shortened time to progression and a lower rate of complete disappearance of neurologic symptoms.

Irradiation is a mainstay of management for patients with intracerebral metastases. Systemic chemotherapy, as of yet, has no clearly defined role in this setting with the exception of corticosteroids (e.g., Dexamethasone) which, when used in high doses (typically 16 mg per day, divided doses) may be acutely effective in relieving associated brain edema.

Among the many possible symptoms produced by intracerebral metastases, headaches, along with motor deficit, disorientation, and seizures, are quite frequent, occurring in 38–55% of all patients studied in large series [25,27]. Radiation therapy is very effective in controlling headache in this context, with 82–93% of patients reporting decrease in pain and 50–55% reporting complete or marked improvement [25,27].

Although survival following the development of brain metastases is typically short (median survivals of four to five months are commonly reported) [24,25,27], there are subsets of patients with decidedly superior prognoses. Favorable factors include ambulatory status, a single brain metastases, brain as the first site of distant metastases, and the presence of headache [27]. Patients with metastases judged suitable for surgical resection in addition to irradiation may fare better than patients managed with irradiation alone, especially patients with single cerebral metastases and minimal systemic tumor burden. In Zimm's series, among 24 such patients managed with surgery and irradiation, the median survival was 10 months with one third alive at one year and 10% alive at 2 years after management. Among 40 patients with a similarly favorable presentation (single cerebral metastases, limited systemic tumor burden) managed with irradiation only, median survival was four months with one- and two-year survivals of 19% and 5%, respectively.

The primary tumors commonly associated with brain metastases include lung (small-cell and non-small-cell variants), breast, malignant melanoma, and hypernephroma. Responses to irradiation are roughly similar irrespective of histology, except by patients with melanoma, who tend to do less well. Katz [28] reported that larger fraction size (≥ 500 cGy) produced a higher rate of response in patients with single cerebral melanoma metastases, but this apparent benefit did not improve duration of response or survival.

With the regimens studied, late radiation effects on the brain have not been prominent, perhaps in part because of the relatively short survivals of these patients as a group and the relatively low total biologic doses administered as compared to doses utilized among patients with primary brain neoplasms. Similarly, the transient deterioration described by Sheline et al. [29] at four to six weeks after irradiation of primary brain neoplasms has not been seen in the palliation of brain metastases. Young et al. [22] reported acute deterioration including death (within hours) when palliation was attempted with 1500 cGy in two fractions among six patients with metastases of choriocarcinoma, testicular carcinoma, or melanoma, but not among patients with metastases from lung or breast cancer. This deterioration occurred in spite of the use of corticosteroids, and was attributed to acute radiation necrosis with hemorrhage among these rapidly growing tumor types. This pattern of deterioration was *not* seen after 1000 cGy in one fraction or 1200 cGy in two fractions in the RTOG study reported by Borgelt et al. [26]. However, in the RTOG study, the number of patients with metastases from choriocarcinoma, testicular carcinoma, or melanoma is not stated.

CHEMOTHERAPY AND HORMONAL THERAPY

Close attention to the previously mentioned general considerations is important for the optimal use of chemotherapeutic agents and hormonal maneuvers (systemic therapy) in the management of cancer-related pain. A thorough understanding of the basic disease, insight into the particular aspects of the individual patient, and an accurate estimate of the overall prognosis with establishment of clear-cut cure or palliative goals all help facilitate the most optimal use of systemic approaches. When systemic therapy is being considered as palliative treatment for pain control, we must ask ourselves a number of questions before proceeding:

1) Would a localized treatment approach be advisable before initiating systemic treatment? For example, a patient with multiple myeloma and a painful lytic lesion

in the humerus with impending fracture would be well served by prophylactic pinning and localized radiotherapy in addition to systemic therapy. Not only would surgical rod placement and local radiotherapy direct intensive treatment to the area of concern, but it would also provide immediate bone stability and minimize pain due to mechanical weakening of the bone.

2) Is the cancer in question sensitive enough to systemic treatment to expect relief of painful symptoms? For example, an elderly woman with painful bone metastases from estrogen-receptor-positive breast cancer is relatively likely to have improvement in bone pain from a hormonal approach. In contrast, a patient with non-small-cell lung cancer metastatic to bone is relatively unlikely to experience substantial pain relief from systemic chemotherapy. Therefore, maximal use of other modalities should be optimized before proceeding with chemotherapy.

3) Are the side effects and toxicities from the proposed therapy worse than the problems from the disease itself? For example, in the management of non-small-cell lung cancer, some patients may experience a period of time, especially early in their course, during which time they are only minimally symptomatic. The use of aggressive, multidrug chemotherapy in such patients will have little if any impact upon survival, yet will severely influence the quality of their life due to drug-related toxicities. The control of pain in such patients would be better done with other modalities since chemotherapy would be relatively unlikely to help. Early initiation of chemotherapy in such a patient would be of little value.

4) Are investigational drugs likely to provide more significant palliation than standard chemotherapy drugs? It is unrealistic for patients or physicians to expect that treatments with drugs in phase I/II stages of evaluation are likely to result in substantial tumor regression and pain relief. Although clinical trials are critically important in the development of new chemotherapy agents, the chances of an individual patient receiving significant antitumor effect in such a clinical trial is unlikely. Consequently, if pain relief is a major goal of treatment, other pain-control measures should be optimized first, rather than relying solely on an investigational drug.

5) What is the optimal timing of systemic intervention? When faced with a diagnosis of incurable cancer, some patients feel an urgency to begin treatment as soon as possible. This "doctor, do something" emotion may be even more prominent in family members. Thus, it may be hard for patients to accept a period of observation of the tumor to assess its pace and overall level of aggressiveness. Some cancers are relatively indolent and/or relatively asymptomatic and can be observed off treatment for many months, avoiding unnecessary toxicity. For example, a patient with minimally symptomatic metastatic prostate cancer may be best served by a period of observation to assess the pace of disease and need for systemic palliative treatment. Although hormonal treatment can provide pain relief, it does not appear to prolong survival. Consequently, its use would most appropriately be reserved for truly symptomatic disease, thus limiting treatment-related side effects. Pain control in such patients might be best managed with other modalities rather than early initiation of hormonal therapy.

6) Have we chosen the least toxic systemic treatment? Some tumors can be palliated just as effectively with minimal therapy as with more aggressive, multi-drug regimens. For example, patients with symptomatic nodular lymphoma may be treated with single-drug chemotherapy with results comparable to those attained with combination chemotherapy [30]. Toxicity is minimized with comparable palliative effect.

Drug scheduling and routes of administration

Changes in drug scheduling may improve chemotherapeutic effect and minimize toxicity. For example, the use of 5-Fluorouracil (5FU) as a continuous systemic infusional agent improves its effect against colorectal and refractory breast cancers and minimizes its toxicity, thereby improving its overall therapeutic index [31,32]. Consequently, it becomes a very useful palliative systemic approach as treatment for colorectal and breast cancers; studies to evaluate its role as palliation for other gastrointestinal tumors and prostate cancer are underway. Likewise, the use of doxorubicin as a protracted infusion as opposed to intermittent bolus therapy may retain its antineoplastic activity yet minimize the degree of nausea, vomiting, anorexia, and cardiac toxicity [33–35].

The use of regional chemotherapy infusion techniques may potentially improve palliative effects with fewer systemic side effects. For example, in selected patients with large, painful unresectable colorectal metastases confined to the liver, the use of regional infusion chemotherapy may provide more rapid and significant relief of pain than systemic therapy [36,37]. Furthermore, patients progressing on systemic therapy can sometimes receive further benefit from infusional therapy directly into the liver.

Patients with leptomeningeal tumor (carcinomatous meningitis) can be treated either with irradiation (cranial, craniospinal), intrathecal chemotherapy, or combined cranial irradiation and intrathecal chemotherapy. Occasionally patients with leptomeningeal tumor can also be treated with certain systemic approaches, such as high-dose ARA-C [38], but in general, direct administration of drug into the cerebrospinal fluid via either spinal tap or preferably Ommaya reservoir provides a more direct, simpler, and less toxic approach to treatment of this isolated metastatic site with chemotherapy [39].

Malignancies where chemotherapy is more likely to prolong life than to provide cure (disseminated cancer of breast or ovary, advanced-stage aggressive lymphoma, extensive smal-cell lung cancer)

In these groups of diseases, chemotherapy may be reasonably expected to provide significant antitumor effect (table 4-4A). Some of these patients may be potentially cured, although most will experience temporary clinical remissions (weeks to months) followed by relapse. Multidrug chemotherapy usually provides increased response rates compared with single drug treatment with more prolongation of survival, but also more toxicity. Consequently, the physician and patient must

61

Table 4-4A. Examples of malignancies where chemotherapy
is likely to significantly prolong life, but unlikely to provide cure

Malignancy	Response Rate	Median Duration of Response	Reference
Nodular lymphomas	>90%	>36 months	(30)
Acute leukemia (adult)	70%	15 months	(50)
Ovarian cancer	60–90%	10–15 months	(40)
Breast cancer	50–70%	9 months	(41)
Small-cell lung cancer (disseminated)	50–70%	6 months	(51)

balance the potential for improved benefit versus the increased toxicity. For example, in the treatment of ovarian cancer, platinum-based chemotherapy regimens are clearly more toxic and inconvenient than single-agent alkylating drugs. However, such combination regimens do provide better response rates with improved survival, and occasionally patients will have significant antitumor effect that is durable from months to years [40]. A reasonable approach would then be to use our best (unfortunately, usually the more toxic) regimens as initial treatment. If it becomes clear that the response is only partial or that only stabilization of disease is achieved, changing to alternative, less toxic, and less frequent chemotherapeutic regimens may be appropriate.

Sometimes in the treatment of such diseases, substantial choice exists about which regimens might be utilized. For example, in the chemotherapeutic treatment of breast cancer, doxorubicin-containing regimens result in comparable survival results compared to non-doxorubicin-containing treatment [41,42]. However, doxorubicin-containing regimens are, in general, more toxic. In patients where metastatic breast cancer is confined to bone and the pace of the disease is relatively slow, the use of a non-doxorubicin-containing regimen at lower doses with less frequent intervals may provide adequate palliation of pain with less toxicity.

Diseases where chemotherapy is relatively unlikely to provide significant prolongation of life (cancers of the gastrointestinal tract, prostate, brain, upper aerodigestive tract, sarcomas)

In this group of diseases, response rates tend to be relatively low and impact on survival rather minimal (table 4-4B). Escalation of drug dosages and use of combination regimens in more aggressive, mutlidrug programs have sometimes resulted in purported increased response rates in small series. However, such results are often not substantiated in larger groupwide studies. Consequently, the beneficial effect of more intensive treatment is uncertain in these diseases. For many such patients, the use of a single chemotherapeutic agent carefully selected and administered in the most toxicity-*limiting* manner is appropriate. If no response occurs, escalation to a more complicated and/or toxic treatment schedule may then be considered. For example, outpatient weekly methotrexate may provide the same

Table 4-4B. Examples of malignancies where chemotherapy is relatively unlikely to provide significant prolongation of life but may palliate symptoms

Malignancy	Response Rate	Median Duration of Response	Reference
Gastrointestinal cancers	15–40%	4–7 months	31, 52
Lung cancer (non-small-cell)	10–30%	2–7 months	53
Upper aerodigestive tract	30–50%	4 months	43
Prostate cancer	10–30%[a]	3–12 months	54
Sarcomas	20–40%	6 months	55
Melanoma	10–20%	4–5 months	56
Brain tumors	—	(time to progression) 6–9 months	57

[a] Response rates for prostate cancer may be reported higher if stable disease category included.

degree of useful palliation for head and neck cancer patients as more toxic, complicated, platinum-based regimens [43]. Treatment goals for this large group of patients are strictly palliative.

Hormonal therapy

The use of hormonal therapies in selected, hormonally responsive cancers provides a potentially ideal, palliative treatment. In general, hormonal therapies have fewer side effects than chemotherapy, may provide excellent relief of pain, and sometimes provide very durable responses. In general, when attempting palliative treatment with a hormonal maneuver, if there is a documented response or period of disease stabilization, a second-line hormonal maneuver may be attempted when progression following the first hormonal treatment is observed. This is especially true in breast cancer where second and third hormonal responses may sometimes be seen. In contrast, second-line responses in prostate and endometrial cancer are unusual. In general, if there is no response to the initial hormonal maneuver, manipulation with a second hormonal approach is unlikely to provide significant benefit.

Breast cancer

Selection of patients who are likely to respond to hormonal maneuvers is best made by the presence of estrogen and progesterone receptors at the time of initial breast biopsy or biopsy of subsequent metastases (table 4-5) [44,45]. Patients most likely to respond to hormonal maneuvers are those whose tumors are both estrogen- and progesterone-receptor positive. In contrast, estrogen-receptor-negative tumors are unlikely to respond. In the absence of estrogen receptor information, other prognostically favorable predictors for response to hormonal maneuvers include older age, bone-predominant metastases, interval of greater than two years from mastectomy to first recurrence, and response to previous hormonal therapy. Therapeutic options for premenopausal women include tamoxifen or oophorectomy. If response occurs, possible subsequent, hormonal maneuvers at the time of

Table 4-5. Response of breast cancers to hormonal manipulation—correlation with receptor status[a]

Receptors	Objective Response
ER − PGR −	10/102 = 10%
ER + PGR −	26/92 = 28%
ER + PGR +	83/109 = 76%

[a] Reference 44, 45.

disease progression include progesterones, androgens, hypophysectomy, and/or adrenalectomy. Adrenalectomy may be performed surgically or medically [41]. In the postmenopausal setting, both exogenous estrogens and tamoxifen have produced comparable response rates. However, tamoxifen is less toxic than estrogens in an elderly population, and clearly would be the preferred treatment. Second-line hormonal approaches include progesterones, androgens, hypophysectomy, and adrenalectomy.

Prostate cancer

Traditional hormonal approaches in the treatment of prostate cancer have been orchiectomy or administration of exogenous estrogens, usually in the form of diethylstilbesterol 1–5 mg/day. Both treatment options produce comparable palliative effects with relief of bone pain in approximately 85% of patients with a median duration of about 15 months. However, neither treatment increases survival [46]. Surgical castration may have undesirable psychological effects, and exogenous estrogens increase the risk of cardiovascular morbidity. If exogenous estrogens are to be administered, prophylactic breast irradiation is useful for preventing gynecomastia which may otherwise be both uncomfortable and disfiguring. Generally, only three to four fractions (treatments) are required. A newer, alternative approach for disseminated prostate cancer is to use gonadotropin-releasing hormone analogues. These drugs inhibit pituitary release of gonadotropins and result in a decrease in testicular steroidogenesis. A prospective randomized trial showed that one such agent, leuprolide, was as effective as diethylstilbesterol (3 mg/day) in the palliation of metastatic prostate cancer and produced fewer side effects [47]. Studies are currently underway to further evaluate the relative role of these newer modality treatments as initial therapy and/or as salvage treatments.

Endometrial cancer

Analagous to breast cancer, endometrial cancer is sometimes hormonally responsive. Traditionally, progestational hormones have been utilized [48], but other hormones such as tamoxifen may be efficacious [49]. The overall response rate to hormonal treatment is approximately 30%. Predictors of hormonal response include the presence of progesterone receptors, well-differentiated histology, and a long disease-free interval from the time of hysterectomy to recurrence.

BIBLIOGRAPHY

1. DeVita VT, Hellman S, Rosenberg SA (eds) (1985): Cancer, Principles and Practice of Oncology, 2nd edition. Philadelphia: Lippincott.
2. Fletcher GH (ed) (1980): Textbook of Radiotherapy, 3rd edition Philadelphia: Lea & Febiger.
3. Moss WT, Brand WN, Battifura H (eds) (1979): Radiation Oncology—Rationale, Techniques, Result, 5th edition. St. Louis: C.V. Mosby.

REFERENCES

1. Ellis F (1969): Dose, time and fractionation: A clinical hypothesis. Clin Radiol 20:1–7.
2. Orton CG, Ellis F (1973): A simplification in the use of the NSD concept in practical radiotherapy. Br J Radiol 46:529–537.
3. Cox JD (1985): Large-dose fractionation (hypo fractionation). Cancer 55:2105–2111.
4. Bosch A (1984): Radiotherapy. In: Twycross RG (ed), Pain Relief in Cancer. Clin Oncol 3:43–57.
5. Richter MP, Coia LR (1985): Palliative radiation therapy. Sem Oncol 12:375–383.
6. Mauch PM, Drew MA (1985): Treatment of metastic cancer to bone. In: DeVita VT, Hellman S, Rosenberg SA (eds), Cancer, Principles and Practice of Oncology, 2nd edition. Philadelphia: Lippincott, chapter 56, section 4, pp 2132–2140.
7. Hendrikson FR, Shehata WM, Kirchner AB (1976): Radiation therapy for osseous metastases. Int J Rad Oncol Biol Phys 1:275–278.
8. Tong D, Gillick L, Hendrickson FR (1982): The palliation of symptomatic osseous metastases—final results of the study by the Radiation Therapy Oncology Group. Cancer 50:893–899.
9. Allen KL, Johnson TW, Hibbs GG (1976): Effective bone palliation as related to various treatment regimens. Cancer 37:984–987.
10. Blitzer PH (1985): Re-analysis of the RTOG study of the palliation of symptomatic osseous metastasis. Cancer 55:1468–1472.
11. Fitzpatrick PD, Rider WD (1976): Half body radiotherapy. Int J Radiat Oncol Biol Phys 1:197–207.
12. Salazar OM, Rubin P, Keller B, Scarantino C (1978): Systemic (half-body) radiation therapy: Response and toxicity. Int J Radiat Oncol Biol Phys 4:937–950.
13. Epstein LM, Stewart BH, Antunez AR, et al. (1979): Half and total body radiation for carcinoma of the prostate. J Urol 122:330–332.
14. Jaffee J, Bosch A, Raich PC (1979): Sequential hemi-body radiotherapy in advanced multiple myeloma. Cancer 43:124–128.
15. Qasim MM (1981): Half body irradiation (HBI) in metastatic carcinomas. Clin Radiol 32:215–219.
16. Nag S, Shah V (1986) Once-a-week lower hemibody irradiation (HBI) for metastatic cancers. Int J Radiat Oncol Biol Phys 12:1003–1005.
17. Salazar OM, Rubin P, Hendrickson Fr, et al. (1986): Single-dose half-body irradiation for palliation of multiple bone metastases from solid tumors. Cancer 58:29–36.
18. Prasad B, Lee M-S, Hendrickson FR (1977): Irradiation of hepatic metastases. Int J Radiat Oncol Biol Phys 2:129–132.
19. Sherman DM, Weichselbaum RW, Order SE, et al. (1978): Palliation of hepatic metastases. Cancer 41:2013–2017.
20. Borgelt BB, Gelber R, Brady LW, et al. (1981): The palliation of hepatic metastases: Results of the Radiation Therapy Oncology Group pilot study. Int J Radiat Oncol Biol Phys 7:589–591.
21. Kinsella TJ (1983): The role of radiation therapy alone and combined with infusion chemotherapy for treating liver metastases. Sem Oncol 10:215–222.
22. Young DF, Posner JB, Chu F, Nisce L (1974): Rapid course radiation therapy of cerebral metastases: Results and complications. Cancer 34:1069–1076.
23. Hendrikson FR (1975): Radiation therapy of metastic tumors. Sem Oncol 2:34–46.
24. Hendrikson FR (1977): The optimum schedule for palliative radiotherapy for metastatic brain cancer. Int J Radiat Oncol Biol Phys 2:165–168.
25. Borgelt B, Gelber R, Kramer S, et al. (1980): The palliation of brain metastases: Final results of the first two studies by the Radiation Therapy Oncology Group. Int J Radiat Oncol Biol Phys 6:1–9.
26. Borgelt B, Gelber R, Larson M, et al. (1981): Ultra-rapid high dose irradiation schedules for the palliation of brain metastases: Final results of the first two studies by the Radiation Therapy Oncology Group. Int J Radiat Oncol Biol Phys 7:1633–1638.

27. Zimm S, Wampler GL, Stablein D, et al. (1981): Intracerebral metastases in solid-tumor patients: Natural history and results of treatment. Cancer 48:384–394.
28. Katz HR (1981): The relative effectiveness of radiation therapy, corticosteroids, and surgery in the management of melanoma metastatic to the central nervous system. Int J Radiat Oncol Biol Phys 7:897–906.
29. Sheline GE, Wara WM, Smith V (1980): Therapeutic irradiation and brain injury Int J Radiat Oncol Biol Phys 6:1215–1228.
30. Portlock CS, Rosenberg SA, Glatstein E (1976): Treatment of advanced non-Hodgkin's lymphoma with favorable histologies. Blood 47:747–756.
31. Quebbeman E, Ausman R, Hansen R, et al. (1985): Long-term ambulatory treatment of metastatic colorectal adenocarcinoma by continuous intravenous infusion of 5-fluorouracil. J Surg Oncol. 30:60–65.
32. Hansen RM, Quebbeman E, Ritch P, et al. (1986): Continuous 5-Flourouracil (5FU) infusion in refractory carcinoma of the breast. Clin Res 34:931A.
33. Legha S, Benjamin R, Mackay B, et al. (1982): Reduction of doxorubicin cardiotoxicity by prolonged continuous intravenous infusion. Ann Intern Med 96:133–139.
34. Lokich J, Bothe A, Zipoli T, et al. (1983): Constant infusion schedule for adriamycin: A phase I-II clinical trial of a 30-day schedule by ambulatory pump delivery system. J Clin Oncol 1:24–8.
35. Garnick MB, Weiss GR, Steele GD, et al. (1983): Clinical evaluation of long-term, continuous infusion doxorubicin. Cancer Treat Rep 67:133–42.
36. Lokich JJ, Ensminger W (1983): Ambulatory pump infusion devices for hepatic artery infusion. Sem Oncol 10:183–190.
37. Oberfield RA (1983): Intra-arterial hepatic infusion chemotherapy in metastatic liver cancer. Sem Oncol 10:206–214.
38. Frick J, Ritch PS, Hansen LM, et al. (1984): Successful treatment of meningeal leukemia using systemic high-dose cytosine arabinoside. J Clin Oncol 5:365–368.
39. Wasserstum W, Glass J, Posner J (1982): Diagnosis and treatment of leptomeningeal metastases from solid tumors. Cancer 49:759–772.
40. Richardson GS, Scully RE, Nikrui N, Nelson J (1985): Common epithelial cancer of the ovary. N Engl J Med 312:415–424, 474–483.
41. Henderson C, Canellos GP (1980): Cancer of the breast. N Engl J Med 302:17–30, 78–90.
42. Brincker H, Rose C, van der Masse H (1984): A randomized study of CAF + TAM (tamoxifen) versus CMF + TAM in metasatic breast cancer. Proc Am Soc Clin Oncol 3:113.
43. Hong WI, Bromer R (1983): Chemotherapy in head and neck cancers. N Engl J Med 308:75–78.
44. McGuire WL (1980): Steroid hormone receptors in breast cancer treatment strategy. Rec Prog Hor Res 36:135–156.
45. Clark GM, McGuire WL (1983): Progesterone receptors in human breast cancer. Breast Cancer Res Treat 3:157–163.
46. Byar DP (1973): Veterans Administration Cooperative Urological Research Group: Studies of cancer of the prostate. Cancer 32:1126–1132.
47. Leuprolid Study Group (1984): Leuprolide versus diethylstilbesterol for metasatic prostate cancer. N Engl J Med 311:1281–1286.
48. Malkasian GD, Decker DG, Mussey E, et al. (1971): Progestin treatment of recurrent endometrical carcinoma. Am J Obstet Gynecol 110:15–21.
49. Swenerton K, Shaw D, White G, Boyer D (1979): Treatment of advanced endometrial carcinoma with tamoxifen. N Engl J Med 301:105.
50. Gale RP (1984): Progress in acute myelogenous leukemia. Ann Intern Med 101: 702–705.
51. Livingston RB, Moore TN, Heilbrun L, et al. (1978): Small-cell carcinoma of the lung: Combined chemotherapy and radiation. Ann Intern Med 88:194–199.
52. Schein PS (1985): The role of chemotherapy in the management of gastric and pancreatic carcinomas. Semin Oncol 12:49–60.
53. Minna JD, Higgins GA, Glatstein EJ (1985): Cancer of the lung. In: DeVita VT, Hellman S, Rosenberg SA (eds), Cancer, Principles and Practice of Oncology, 2nd edition. Philadelphia: Lippincott, chapter 18, pp 558–564.
54. Torti FM, Carter SK (1980): The chemotherapy of prostatic adenocarcinoma. Ann Intern Med 92:681–689.
55. Rosenberg SA, Suit HD, Baker LH (1985): Sarcomas of soft tissues. In: DeVita VT, Hellman S,

Rosenberg SA (eds), Cancer, Principles and Practice of Oncology, 2nd edition. Philadelphia: Lippincott, chapter 36, pp 1279–1283.
56. Mastrangelo MJ, Baker AR, Katz HR (1985): Cutaneous melanoma. In: DeVita VT, Hellman S, Rosenberg SA (eds), Cancer, Principles and Practice of Oncology, 2nd edition. Philadelphia: Lippincott, chapter 39, pp 1404–1406.
57. Kornblith PL, Walker MD, Cassady JR (1985): Neoplasms of the central nervous system. In: DeVita VT, Hellman S, Rosenberg SA (eds), Cancer, Principles and Practice of Oncology, 2nd edition. Philadelphia: Lippincott, chapter 41, pp 1471–1481.

5. THE ROLE OF NONNEUROLYTIC NERVE BLOCKS IN THE MANAGEMENT OF CANCER PAIN

STEPHEN E. ABRAM, M.D.

The approach to the management of cancer pain should generally be a progression from relatively low-risk, noninvasive techniques, to modalities that are somewhat more invasive, cause some discomfort and carry a somewhat higher risk, to high-risk, invasive procedures, which are generally reserved for desperate situations. Oral analgesics, psychotropics, and nonsteroid anti-inflammatory drugs are the usual first-line treatment for patients with cancer pain. Prior to consideration of more invasive techniques, we must insure that adequate doses of appropriate analgesics and adjuvant drugs have been tried. Approximately one third of our referrals for neurolytic blocks or intraspinal narcotics respond promptly to adjustment of their oral medications.

If the patient does not obtain sufficient pain relief from analgesic agents or exhibits somnolence or major side effects from otherwise adequate doses, then somewhat more involved procedures must be considered. Unfortunately, the next step is too often the use of neurodestructive blocks or surgery. A substantial number of patients benefit dramatically from techniques that modulate neural responses to noxious stimuli. These techniques include local anesthetic nerve blocks, intraspinal narcotics, transcutaneous and percutaneous nerve stimulation techniques, and a number of cognitive strategies (hypnosis, distraction, biofeedback). This discussion will concentrate primarily on applications of nonneurolytic nerve blocks utilizing local anesthetics and/or corticosteroids.

Nondestructive nerve blocks have two major functions: therapy for intractable pain and prognostic/diagnostic function. The therapeutic uses of nerve blocks include treatment of sympathetically mediated pain syndromes (causalgia, reflex sympathetic dystrophy), muscle infiltration for myofascial pain, perineural steroid injection for neuropathic conditions, control of severe acute pain (rib fracture, postoperative pain, acute Herpes Zoster) and temporary relief of incapacitating pain. Nerve blocks are used diagnostically to differentiate between visceral and somatic pain, or between sympathetically mediated pain and somatic pain. They may also be used diagnostically to demonstrate a particular neural pathway involved with a patient's pain. Prognostic blocks are used to predict the efficacy of subsequent neurodestructive procedures.

CAUSALGIA AND REFLEX SYMPATHETIC DYSTROPHY

Reflex sympathetic dystrophy (RSD) is a syndrome characterized by pain, often burning in quality, sensory distortion (hyperesthesia, hyperpathia, allodynia), autonomic instability in the affected area (warm, flushed skin or cool, cyanotic skin, edema, hyperhydrosis) and, later in its course, dystrophic changes (smooth, glossy skin, joint stiffness and swelling, bone demineralization, muscle atrophy). Most cases in the general population are posttraumatic or postoperative. Suspicion that the condition exists is raised when pain is more severe than would be expected for the degree of injury or when pain outlasts the usual recovery period. It is a condition that is easily overlooked or forgotten in the cancer patient, who is expected to have pain. Among cancer patients, it may be triggered by surgery, radiation, tumor spread or pathological fracture.

Causalgia is similar to RSD in symptomatology, but is, by definition, associated with major nerve injury. Most reported cases are caused by gunshot wounds, and most involve injury to nerves proximal to the knee or the elbow [1]. The median nerve, medial cord of the brachial plexus or the tibial division of the sciatic nerve are the neural structures most often injured in cases of causalgia, perhaps because they have high populations of sympathetic fibers projecting to the palm of the hand and sole of the foot [2].

Several theories have been proposed to explain sympathetically mediated pain. A simple reflex increase in sympathetic activity, triggered by painful stimulation and leading to vasoconstriction, ischemia, and more painful stimulation, is one of the older explanations. Although it is far too simplistic, that explanation may have some merit. Alterations is sympathetic function have been demonstrated following peripheral nerve lesions in animals [3]. Short-circuiting of efferent sympathetic discharges across injured nerve segments may be capable of activating afferent nociceptor fibers. Although there is anatomic evidence that loss of insulating myelin or Schwann-cell sheaths does occur, there is little physiologic evidence for ephaptic transmission [4].

Injured peripheral nerves often differ from normal fibers physiologically: they fire spontaneously, they become very sensitive to mechanical stimulation, and they increase their firing in response to sympathetic nerve activity or locally applied catecholamines [5,6]. Devor [4] suggests that these acquired characteristics of injured nerves are related to the appearance of large numbers of inward-conducting sodium and calcium channels and adrenergic receptors on the nerve sprout or injured nerve segment.

Although sympathetic nervous system activity has not been shown to alter sensitivity of nociceptors, it does increase sensitivity of some mechanoreceptors [7]. Roberts [7] proposed that the pain on light touch so often seen in RSD may be related to a combination of sympathetically induced mechanoreceptor sensitivity plus sensitization of wide-dynamic-range neurons in the dorsal horn.

Local anesthetic block of the sympathetic chain is the usual initial treatment of reflex sympathetic dystrophy. In relatively acute cases, it is often the only therapy required. The initial block usually produces analgesia that outlasts the local anesthetic duration. Subsequent injections, given daily or every other day, produce gradual resolution of symptoms. Several injections are usually required before symptoms disappear permanently. In chronic cases, in which dystrophic changes are severe, extensive physical rehabilitation is the most important aspect of treatment, but sympathetic blocks may help provide analgesia to facilitate physical therapy. Causalgia is more resistant to treatment than RSD. Surgical sympathectomy is generally regarded to be the proper treatment for this condition, although some cases can be successfully managed with aggressive nerve block therapy [8].

RSD that occurs in cancer patients may be more resistant to treatment than cases that occur after trauma. If the condition was triggered by tumor invasion of soft tissues or nerves, it is likely that the condition will recommence after therapy is stopped. Nevertheless, many patients will experience many days or sometimes weeks of relief followng sympathetic blocks, and pain can sometimes be adequately controlled by performing blocks at intervals of one to several weeks. RSD in cancer patients that is triggered by surgery rather than tumor or pathological fracture may respond dramatically and permanently to nerve block therapy.

Intravenous regional administration of guanethidine has been advocated as an alternative means of achieving sympathetic blockade. The technique has been shown to be as effective as local anesthetic block for treating RSD of nonmalignant origin [9]. It has the advantage of being safe for patients with coagulopathies, but is not likely to be of benefit if pain is in the proximal portions of the limb. We found that patients who experienced transient relief from sympathetic blocks (minutes to hours) were likely to get more prolonged relief with intravenous regional guanethidine block (one to several days), but were unlikely to experience long-term or permanent relief [10].

It is not clear whether burning pain and hyperpathia associated with damage by tumor to the brachial or femoral plexus should be called a true causalgia. Semantics aside, such problems are generally more resistant to treatment with local anesthetic sympathetic blocks. If, in such cases, sympathetic blocks produce profound but temporary relief, continuous blocking techniques, such as continuous epidural or continuous brachial plexus block, carried out for a period of several days, may produce lasting relief. If not, neurolytic or surgical sympathectomy might be considered. If sympathetic block produces no relief, even temporarily, then further sympathetic intervention is not warranted.

HERPES ZOSTER

Acute herpes zoster infection and postherpetic neuralgia are common pain disorders among patients with malignancy. There is at least anecdotal evidence that sympathetic blocks, performed early in the course of the disease, may relieve symptoms, hasten disappearance of the rash, and prevent or at least diminish the severity of post-herpetic neuralgia. Unfortunately, the paucity of controlled studies of the efficacy of such treatment precludes concluding that sympathetic blocks alter the course of the disease. By the same token, we are unable to say conclusively that the technique is worthless.

A patient we treated with severe acute herpes zoster illustrates the type of response to sympathetic blocks that convinces many practitioners of the benefit of this therapy. A thirty-year-old woman had stage 3 Hodgkin's disease and a five-day history of unilateral mid-thoracic pain and exquisite hyperpathia. She had a rash composed of confluent, weeping vesicles which covered the entire T-8 and T-9 dermatomes on the right. Her pain was not affected at all by Percodan. A single-shot epidural was administered in the low thoracic region, just below the level of the rash, using 10 ml 3% chloroprocaine to achieve sympathetic and somatic blockade. The procedure produced complete relief lasting several hours. The pain recurred for several hours but dissipated gradually over the next several hours. By the next day the patient was pain-free and the vesicles had begun to dry. Her subsequent recovery was prompt and uneventful.

There is no way of knowing whether this patient would have recovered promptly without treatment. Whether local anesthetic blockade promotes healing of the pathological process or not, it certainly provides profound analgesia during the acute phase. For lesions above T-4, stellate ganglion blocks will provide at least temporary relief. For lesions at or below T-4, continuous epidural blockade with dilute concentrations of anesthetic will provide excellent comfort without motor block. Blocks are usually continued until the herpetic vesicles begin to dry and clear.

MYOFASCIAL PAIN

Myofascial syndrome is a common painful disorder characterized by tender, spontaneously painful foci in muscles, known as trigger points. These pressure-sensitive trigger points are often found in tight, ropey bands of muscle. Mechanical stimulation of a trigger point produces local pain plus referred pain, whose distribution is characteristic of the involved muscle. While the pathophysiology is not entirely clear, there are some theories regarding pain mechanisms. Travell and Simons [11] propose that acute muscle strain leads to tissue damage with tearing of the sarcoplasmic reticulum and calcium release. The excess local calcium causes sustained or repeated contraction followed by increased metabolism, reduced perfusion, and fatigue. ATP depletion prevents release of myosin from actin, causing sarcomeres to become rigid at that length. The muscle becomes taut. Release of vasoactive peptides and amines from platelets and mast cells causes sensitization of muscle afferents, leading to pain and mechanosensitivity.

Cancer patients often develop myofascial pain, which is probably most often secondary to somatic or visceral pain from the spread of their tumor. Reflex muscle spasm caused by bony, neural, or visceral pain leads to the sequence of events described above. Trigger-point injections with local anesthetic may be surprisingly effective in the patient's overall pain management. When summation of myofascial inputs plus other visceral or somatic afferent inputs causes perception of pain, reduction of the muscle afferent activity may be enough to provide profound relief. Repeated injections carried out every several days for a week or two may produce lasting benefit. Vapocoolant spray (Fluori-methane) of the trigger points followed by gentle mobilization and stretching of the involved muscle may be a helpful adjunct. Transcutaneous electrical stimulation of the trigger points may also provide some relief.

NEUROPATHIC PAIN

Invasion or compression of intraspinal nerve roots, brachial and femoral plexus, or major peripheral nerves is a source of severe pain in cancer patients. Mechanical compression of major neural structures may induce a chronic inflammatory process, accompanied by accumulation of serum proteins, an increase in intraneural pressure, ischemia, and eventually a loss of axons [12]. Suspensions of insoluble steroids appear to ameliorate symptoms of lumbar and cervical radiculopathy when injected epidurally, presumably by reducing the inflammatory response of the affected nerve roots [13]. Devor et al. [14] have provided experimental evidence that steroids applied directly to recently injured peripheral nerves can significantly reduce spontaneous activity in afferent nerve fibers. They suggest that the effect is related to a direct membrane action rather than an anti-inflammatory effect.

It is likely that the neural pathology associated with tumor compression is similar to that caused by a herniated or bulging disc. On the basis of the assumption, we have treated a variety of cancer-related neuropathological disorders with perineural injections of local anesthetic and triamcinolone diacetate.

If epidural tumor spread is suspected, an epidural injection of the mixture is carried out. We select triamcinolone diacetate because it mixes easily with local anesthetic without clumping (unlike methylprednisolone acetate) and it has been shown not to cause neurological or meningeal pathology when injected epidurally in animals [15]. A single injection of triamcinolone 50 mg with 5 ml 1% lidocaine is performed. Pain relief within minutes of injection signifies correct placement of the drug mixture with anesthesia of the pathological nerve roots. Pain often recurs as the local anesthetic effect subsides. If the steroid is effective, there will be gradual improvement in symptoms over the next 24 to 72 hours. Duration of analgesia is usually one to four weeks. Repeat injections are usually effective in reestablishing analgesia. We have treated patients for several months with such intermittent injections.

Patients with tumor invasion of the brachial plexus may benefit from brachial plexus blockade with steroid and local anesthetic. The approach used depends on the site of plexus involvement. Pancoast tumors that involve the proximal portions of the plexus are more likely to respond to interscalene or subclavian perivascular approaches. If tumor invasion is closer to the axilla, an infraclavicular or axillary approach may be preferable. Doses are similar to those used for steroid epidurals. Onset and duration of analgesia is also similar to that seen with epidurals. Patients with severe hyperpathia associated with neurological loss may experience profound numbness that was previously masked by the severe burning pain, and should be warned of that possibility, lest the block be blamed for the sensory deficit. Pelvic tumors invading the femoral plexus may also respond to similar therapy. A paravertebral approach to the femoral plexus, the so-called psoas compartment block [16] provides the best approach. The following case report illustrates the potential efficacy of perineural steroid injections.

Case report

The patient is a 33-year-old woman with recurrent squamous cell carcinoma of the cervix. Abdominal and pelvic CT scan two weeks prior to Pain Clinic evaluation showed a large left pelvic tumor invading muscle and other soft tissues of the left lateral pelvic wall. She presented with a two-month history of left buttock and leg pain which radiated to the toes, and weakness of left foot dorsiflexion. Methadone 5 mg bid and Percodan q6h provided incomplete pain relief. The patient slept poorly because of the pain.

Examination revealed pain on straight leg raising to 45 degrees on the left, marked weakness of left foot dorsiflexion, absent sensation through L-5 on the left and absent left ankle jerk.

Initial treatment consisted of an epidural injection of 50 mg triamcinolone diacetate plus 4 ml 1% lidocaine and an L4-5 psoas compartment femoral plexus block with 50 mg triamcinolone diacetate plus 5 ml normal saline. The procedure produced prompt relief of pain. A week later the patient reported that she was nearly pain-free. Five weeks later, the patient returned complaining of some pain recurrence, but her pain was not as severe as before the steroid injections. Both the epidural and psoas compartment blocks were repeated using the same steroid doses. When she returned two weeks later, she had some mild to moderate upper thigh pain. A psoas compartment block was performed at the L4-5 level with 50 mg triamcinolone diacetate and 4 ml 1% lidocaine. That procedure produced two months of near complete pain relief. Residual pain was well controlled with methadone 5 mg b.i.d. and occasional Percodan. During that period of time, she experienced an increase in leg weakness. Subsequent examination demonstrated marked left quadriceps, dorsiflexor, and plantar flexor weakness. Knee and ankle jerks were absent on the left, and there was edema of the entire left leg. Her pain was well controlled for the next four months on stable oral narcotic doses. Subsequent hip pain recurrence was felt to be related to tumor destruction of the acetabulum, and no further nerve block treatment was carried out.

DIAGNOSTIC BLOCKS

Local anesthetic blocks may be useful in assessing mechanisms or pathways of pain perception. It is often useful to determine whether pain is of a somatic or a visceral nature. Comparison of the analgesic effect of a celiac plexus block to the analgesia from a somatic block (paravertebral nerve root block, intercostal block) is useful in assessing whether abdominal pain is of intraperitoneal origin or of body-wall origin. Chest pain that is primarily of a visceral nature responds well to cervicothoracic sympathetic blockade, while chest-wall pain will improve following appropriate intercostal blocks. In performing such diagnostic procedures it is important to perform at least one placebo injection (e.g., intramuscular saline) and to compare the response of diagnostic blocks to the placebo response. If the degree and duration of the placebo injection is similar to that of the local anesthetic blocks, then placebo response to the blocks is likely. If the patient experiences a longer duration or much more profound analgesic response to the nerve block, it is likely that the block produced analgesia because of the neural blockade.

Nerve blocks may also be helpful in determining whether pain in nonvisceral structures has a sympathetic mechanism. If pain is relieved by stellate ganglion block or lumbar sympathetic block, but not by placebo, a significant contribution to the pain by sympathetic mechanisms is likely, and procedures that alter sympathetic function (surgical or chemical sympathectomy, sympathetic blocking drugs) may be of some benefit. Unfortunately, a positive response to local-anesthetic sympathetic block does not necessarily predict long-term benefit from sympathectomy.

The techniques of differential spinal or epidural blockade have been developed to ascertain the mechanism of lower extremity or lower trunk pain [17]. The technique is based on the early observations by Erlanger and Gasser [18] that small nerve fibers are more sensitive to blocking effects of local anesthetics. Subsequent studies by Heavner and de Jong [19] suggested that B fibers (preganglionic autonomics) are more sensitive than small afferent (nociceptive) fibers. Dilute anesthetic solutions should, therefore, be capable of blocking sympathetic fibers while sparing nociceptors. However, single-fiber recording studies have uniformly failed to demonstrate the differential blocking effect of local anesthetics on small vs. large fibers [20,21]. Franz and Perry [20], however, demonstrated that small fibers block more quickly and recover more slowly than large fibers. The technique of *retrograde* spinal or epidural block [17] may, therefore, be a more rational technique. With this technique, normal saline is injected initially. If no placebo response occurs, a motor and sensory blocking concentration of anesthetic is injected, using a dose adequate to completely block all nerves in the affected area. If no pain relief occurs despite profound anesthesia, it is assumed that the pain arises above the level of block (*central or psychogenic pain*). If pain is relieved by the anesthetic, then the observer records the return of sensory and motor function and correlates these observations with the return of pain. If pain returns coincident with the return of sympathetic function (fall in skin temperature), a sympathetic mechanism is assumed to be present. If the return of pain coincides with the return of sensation, and the sympathetic block is still in effect, the mechanism is likely to be somatic, with little or no sympathetic contribution.

PROGNOSTIC BLOCKS

Local anesthetic blocks are often used to predict the efficacy of neuroablative procedures such as chemical or surgical rhizotomy, gasserian ganglion ablation, celiac plexus neurolysis, or sympathectomy. Prognostic blocks also allow the patient to experience the sensory loss that will accompany loss of neural function, so they are better equipped to decide about accepting the procedure. Unfortunately, local anesthetic blocks do not reliably predict the long-term benefit of permanent blocks or surgery. The reason that pain recurs following rhizotomy or neurectomy probably relates to functional changes in dorsal horn neurons, which are ordinarily activated by noxious input (nociceptive-specific and wide-dynamic-range neurons). Following loss of neuronal input to these cells, they regain their previous level of activity or even increase their activity through the following mechanisms: 1) switching on of previously ineffective synapses; 2) increased efficacy of remaining synapses; 3) development of aberrant connections from sprouts from other neurons; and 4) development of chemical supersensitivity of these cells to neurotransmitters released in the vicinity [22]. There is experimental evidence that opiate-mediated suppression of pain-projection cells may be reduced or lost following reduction of afferent input. Lamotte et al [23], for instance, have demonstrated a reduction in the number of opiate receptors in the ipsilateral dorsal horn following unilateral rhizotomy in primates.

Some patients who experience pain relief from sympathetic blocks experience only transient relief from surgical or chemical sympathectomy. The reasons for such failures are still obscure. Some cases undoubtedly represent incomplete sympathectomy. Other cases may be due to postdenervation hypersensitivity of adrenergic receptors in the affected limb, which could be activated by low circulating levels of catecholamines. Oral or intravenous regional sympathetic blocking drugs such as guanethidine or prazosin may be helpful in such patients.

Although an analgesic response to local anesthetic blocks does not necessarily predict a lasting response to neuroablative procedures, a lack of response to local anesthetic blocks does reliably predict failure. It is, therefore, worthwhile to perform predictive nerve blocks whenever a permanent procedure is anticipated.

CRISIS MANAGEMENT

Occasionally, cancer patients will develop such severe, intractable pain that it cannot be controlled with narcotic analgesics without producing complete obtundation. Such severe pain may rapidly lead to psychological decompensation. The temporary use of continuous local anesthetic blocks, such as continuous epidural or continuous brachial plexus block, can provide complete analgesia without affecting mental function. The profound analgesia will have a salutory effect on psychological status, and will permit reduction in narcotic doses, allowing time to reverse some of the tolerance which has developed. Such drug holidays are useful for patients who have developed extreme tolerance to epidural narcotics. Continuous infusion of 0.125% bupivacaine will generally provide good analgesia without profound motor block. Local anesthetic toxicity does not appear to be a problem with bupivacaine if the dose is limited to 30 mg/hr, even in patients whose drug clearance is reduced by renal or hepatic disease [24]. Some cancer patients develop high serum levels of bupivacaine without signs of systemic toxicity. The phenomenon appears to be related to high levels of alpha-acid glycoprotein, a plasma protein fraction that binds much of the circulating bupivacaine [24].

REFERENCES

1. Richards RL (1967): Causalgia: A centennial review. Arch Neurol 16.339–350.
2. Sunderland S (1976): Pain mechanisms in causalgia. J Neurol Neurosurg Psychiat 39:471–480.
3. Blumberg H, Janig W (1983): Changes in vasoconstrictor neurons supplying cat hindlimb following chronic nerve lesions: A model for studying mechanisms of reflex sympathetic dystrophy? J Auton Nerv Syst 7:399–411.
4. Devor M (1983): Nerve pathophysiology and mechanisms of pain in causalgia. J Auton Nerv Syst 7:371–384.
5. Wall PD, Gutnick M (1974): Ongoing activity in peripheral nerves: The physiology and pharmacology of impulses originating from a neuroma. Exp Neurol 43:580–593.
6. Devor M, Janig W (1981): Activation of myelinated afferents ending in a neuroma by stimulation of the sympathetic supply in the rat. Neurosci Lett 24:43–47.
7. Roberts WJ (1986): A hypothesis on the physiologic basis for causalgia and related pains. Pain 24:297–311.
8. Bonica JJ (1979): Causalgia and reflex sympathetic dystrophies. In: Bonica JJ, Albe-Fessard D (eds), Advances in Pain Research and Therapy, vol 3. New York: Raven Press, pp 141–166.
9. Boneli S, Conoscente F, Movilla PG, et al. (1983): Regional intravenous guanethidine vs stellate block in reflex sympathetic dystrophies: a randomized trial. Pain 16:297–308.
10. Abram SE, Kettler RE, Reynolds AC, et al. (1986): Potential advantage of IV regional guanethidine over sympathetic blocks. ASRA Abstracts 11:85.
11. Travell JG, Simons DG (1983): Myofascial Pain and Dysfunction. Baltimore: Williams and Wilkins.
12. Murphy RW (1977): Nerve roots and spinal nerves in degenerative disc disease. Clin Orthop 129:46–60.
13. Benzon HT (1986): Epidural steroids for low back pain and lumbosacral radiculopathy. Pain 24:277–295.
14. Devor M, Govrin-Lippmann R, Raber P (1985): Corticosteroids suppress ectopic neural discharge originating in experimental neuromas. Pain 22:127–137.
15. Delaney TJ, Rowlingson JC, Carron HC, et al. (1980): Epidural effects on nerves and meninges. Anesth Analg 59:610–614.
16. Chayen D, Nathan H, Chayen M (1976): The psoas compartment block. Anesthesiology 45:95–99.
17. Raj PP, Ramamurthy S (1986): Differential nerve block studies. In: Raj PP (ed), Practical Management of Pain. Chicago: Year Book, pp 173–177.
18. Gasser HS, Erlanger J (1929): The role of fiber size in the establishment of a nerve block by pressure or cocaine. Am J Physiol 88:581–591.
19. Heavner JE, de Jong RH (1974): Lidocaine blocking concentrations for B- and C-nerve fibers. Anesthesiology 40:228–233.
20. Franz DN, Perry S (1974): Mechanisms for differential block among single myelinated and non-myelinated axons by procaine. J Physiol 236:193–210.
21. Fink BR, Cairns AM (1983): Differential peripheral axon block with lidocaine: unit studies in the cervical vagus nerve. Anesthesiology 59:182–186.
22. Zimmerman M (1979): Peripheral and central nervous mechanisms of nociception, pain and pain therapy: Facts and hypotheses. In: Bonica JJ et al. (eds), Advances in Pain Research and Therapy vol 3. New York: Raven Press, pp 3–32.
23. Lamotte C, Pert CB, Snyder SH (1976): Opiate receptor binding in primate spinal cord: distribution and changes after dorsal root section. Brain Res 112:407–412.
24. Raj PP, Denson DD (1986): Prolonged analgesia technique with local anesthetics. In: Raj PP (ed), Practical Management of Pain. Chicago, Year Book, pp 687–703.

6. INTRASPINAL NARCOTICS FOR INTRACTABLE CANCER PAIN

DENNIS WM. COOMBS, M.D.

Few clinicians would disagree that cancer pain is an important problem, especially when the patient is experiencing or appears to suffer unrelieved agony. Pain may be difficult to relieve for a number of reasons. The clinician must appreciate the major factors leading to intractability in order to place in proper context both the advances as well as the limitations of intraspinal narcotic therapy in cancer pain therapy.

Indeed, most of the technique's potential deficiencies were overlooked during the early enthusiastic adoption of spinal narcotics [1]. Why did this critical scientific lapse occur? First, the ease of institution created a new outlet for the talents of anesthesiologists, many of whom were new to chronic pain therapy. A pervasive clinical optimism fueled this revolution based upon promising research advances in spinal narcotic neuropharmacology. Perhaps there is a moral in this. Animal pain models are essential to progress in pain therapy, but no paradigm yet contrived can duplicate the dynamic temporal complexity of cancer pain. A further factor has been the lack of controlled studies delineating the relative merits of conventional analgesia versus spinal narcotic. Currently, clinicians are without knowledge of the circumstances under which spinal narcotics are either indicated for their intrinsic merits or contraindicated due to side effects of impotency. With this dose of restraint, we will attempt to place in current context the use and limitations of spinal narcotics in the treatment of cancer pain and their relationship to conventional and radical options to

This review was supported in part by U.S. Public Health Service Grant—CA 33865 of the National Cancer Institute and the Robert Osgood Jr. Memorial Fund.

control cancer pain syndromes. Clearly, this subject is too broad for a short monograph to encompass. Thus, only general guidelines and major problem syndromes will be highlighted.

MECHANISMS OF PAIN ASSOCIATED WITH CANCER

This subject has been nicely reviewed recently by Foley [2]. Cancer pain has been described as acute, intermittent acute, and chronic—acute intermittent pain. The syndromes seen include tumor-associated acute pain, cancer-therapy-associated pain, and chronic cancer-related pains either due to cancer therapy or tumor progression. Mechanistically, cancer pain derives from a variety of pathophysiologic processes that give rise to the aforementioned patterns of pain perception. Individually, these processes include compression and invasion of nervous roots, trunks, and plexus; tumor invasion of bone; invasion or obstruction of blood vessels and lymphatics; obstruction and distention of hollow viscus or ductal systems; swelling in encapsulated or ensheathed structures; and inflammatory, ulcerating or necrotic processes [2,3]. One, a few, or all of these processes may occur at any time in variable intensity in any given tumor syndrome, giving rise to both a variety of presentations and dynamic courses. Not surprisingly, therapy must be polymodal and equally dynamic to obtain adequate and sustained results over the long course in many patients. From a neurophysiologic angle, the location of the tumor process leads to a variety of pain presentations whose classification has been found useful both prognostically and therapeutically. Thus cancer and the pathophysiologic processes enumerated above may lead to any or several of the following syndromes: somatic, visceral, neurogenic, deafferentation, and reflex sympathetic pain. Further, the presentation may be acute or intermittently acute-chronic. Finally, it must be remembered that patients may experience procedural or postsurgical pain in addition to common pain syndromes unrelated to the cancer itself, e.g., arthritis, ulcers, angina, and herniated discs. One must be wary not to ascribe all pain to malignancy, thus prematurely giving up the ghost, while realizing that preexisting personality disorders and drug abuse yield extremely complex pain problems to diagnose and manage.

DEPRESSION AND SUFFERING

The cancer pain therapist must deal with a complicated psychoemotional state arising from the terminal nature of cancer processes. Most cancer patients experience at least transient situational depression [4]. Psychological depression is well known to increase the magnitude of pain reporting regardless of the context [5]. Cancer pain crises often correlate with an emotional or depressive nadir for the patient. Thus one of the most effective approaches to such pain is to employ the skills of a psychiatrist experienced in evaluating depression in this setting [6]. This consultation may be beneficial for many reasons: 1) the psychiatric consultant may help diagnostically if mental organicity exists—for example, depression may be part of preexisting organic disease, alcoholism, organic brain syndrome, Alzheimer's, etc.; 2) the

Table 6-1. Alternatives for cancer pain control

Agents/Procedures	Indications/Pain
1. Anti-inflammatories	Bone pain-tumor inflammation
2. Antidepressants (high dose)	Treat depression
Antidepressants (low dose)	For most intractable pain
3. Amphetamine	Overcome narcotic sedation
4. Antiseizure drugs (i.e. carbamazepine)	Deafferentation
5. Calcitonin	Bone pain
6. Local anesthetic injection	Myofascitis, RSD, neurogenic
7. Neurolytics	Neurogenic
8. Hypophysectemy (alcohol)	Generalized pain (i.e., breast, prostate)
9. Neurosury (i.e., cordotomy)	Unilateral lower extremity

consultant may contribute a detoxification plan if analgesic side effects adversely effect therapy of depression or anxiety; 3) psychiatrists are intimately familiar with antidepressants, anxiolytics, and major tranquilizers, some or all of which may be indicated or require detoxification; 4) the psychiatrist may help the struggling patient to adopt more effective coping strategies through relaxation therapy, biofeedback, or simply structured interview; and 5) this consultation may prevent overly aggressive therapies from being interjected by identifying inappropriate pain behavior, preexisting hypochondriacal or hysterical tendencies, or overt psychological deterioration. However, the final responsibility for evaluating difficult and intractable patients resides with the pain specialist in consultation with these ancillary disciplines. Once effective pain control is delivered, many psychological crises abate with emergence of a new, reasonable patient.

EFFECTIVE ANALGESIC POLYPHARMACY

Most cancer pain patients will experience several mechanisms and thus types of pain over their malignant course. Consequently, a variety of analgesic approaches may be required over time. Table 6-1 lists alternative analgesic therapies and some situations in which they are particularly helpful. Alternative strategies are particularly relevant to spinal narcotics for cancer pain because 1) new therapies are often instituted before safe and effective oral and systemic therapies are thoroughly tried; 2) some adjunctive therapies must be instituted or continued in order to achieve good results with spinal narcotics; and 3) adjunctive therapies may need to be halted to eliminate side effects from spinal analgesic coadministration.

Some guidelines regarding these adjunctive or primary agents require emphasis. First, the recent addition of sustained-action oral morphine preparations has substantially reduced the number of truly intractable cancer pain patients seen by our pain service. Several common errors made with oral narcotics in the cancer patient include 1) narcotic dosage and frequency is insufficiently aggressive; 2) physicians rely upon short-acting narcotics, resulting in severe peaks and valleys in analgesic blood levels and often in pronounced sleep disorders; 3) insufficient time is taken to establish proper dose of longer-duration narcotics given their variable drug half-life in cancer patients—methadone is the prime example; and 4) CNS side effects arise frequently either because of long half-life, coadministration of anxiolytics, anti-cholinergic side-effect susceptibility, or psychotomimetic properties of narcotic preparations.

There is no cocktail approach that will work for all patients, but the following basic strategy has served our clinic well. In early pain syndromes, we first institute an anti-inflammatory drug such as ibuprofen. The choice depends upon several factors: overall integrity of excretory systems; gastric susceptibility to NSAIDS or past history of allergy, asthma, nasal polyps, or ulcer; and magnitude of bony involvement of inflammatory processes. Next we institute oxycodone or hydromorphone if the pain is intermittent, in combination with NSAIDS—don't stop these agents. We use acetaminophen if nothing else is acceptable. For more persistent and difficult pain, a morphine preparation is added, preferably MS Contin. Alternatively, Roxanol or other morphine solutions are used. At times hydromorphone, morphine, or oxymorphone suppositories will be needed if PO is impossible. Finally, an antidepressant is almost always helpful if low-dose narcotics and anti-inflammatories together are inadequate. Drugs like amitriptyline at 25–50 mg/day (first choice usually) are analgesic at modest doses, rapidly improve sleep patterns when given HS, and at these doses do not generally yield troublesome side effects in combination with other agents. Serious depression should prompt higher doses, testing for adequate therapeutic blood levels, and the consideration of psychiatric consultation.

The above constitutes a first-stage approach. Failure of these regimens requires a repeat look at the basic mechanisms for the pain so as to better treat and control it. First, serious attempts to control the pain may require aggressive dosage escalation of narcotic. In terminal pain there is no upper dose limit as long as the patients are cognitively intact and still in pain. This may require high-dose oral morphine, sometimes over 1000 mg per day! Alternatively, levo-phanol or methadone is used. In such cases a shorter duration drug, such as hydromorphone, is used q 4–6 Hr for breakthrough pain prophylaxis. Reference to recent reviews on this subject are advised, since 1) there is much that is new on these subjects; and 2) the decision to proceed to spinal narcotics is predicated on the idea that an adequate trial of conventional systemic narcotics has been achieved [7,8]. Alternative approaches have been suggested including the use of continuous subcutaneous or intravenous morphine infusions and recently the use of patient-controlled analgesia systems [9–11]. Their exact place is probably less well defined than spinal narcotics given the dearth of publications and the lack of controlled comparisons.

INTRACTABLE CANCER PAIN

So far, much has been said about the hierarchy of analgesic approaches taken to cancer pain and the classification of syndromes for better therapy. At this point, several biases must be exposed. First, much has been written and said about cancer pain patients who take tremendous doses of narcotics with no apparent impact on cognition. This happens. It also happens that prolonged observation by family and others frequently reveals periods of inattention, nodding, and difficulty focusing on tasks. Some patients display subtle changes in wit and personality. This is not surprising since opiate receptors are widely and densely represented throughout the limbic system and neocortex [12]. Opioid receptor tolerance is not complete within dose ranges usually achieved. Further, incomplete cross-reactivity occurs at other opioid receptor subtypes (kappa, delta, etc.) with agonists considered to be predominately mu-selective. To this extent, narcotic approaches that understimulate supraspinal opioid receptors, such as continuous spinal opiate analgesia, appear to have less impact on rostral cerebral opioid receptors [13]. This has been suggested by the lack of drug reward seeking in animal models comparing spinal and supraspinal narcotic delivery (recently challenged) [14]. Finally, spinal drugs with prolonged activity, such as morphine, parallel the advantages of sustained-release oral narcotics without their adverse actions. This is particularly important when complex pain syndromes are encountered requiring the coadministration of adjunctive agents and narcotic by whatever route or when drug elimination problems exist.

INTRACTABILITY

The efficacy of spinal narcotic analgesia is not at issue (see several excellent reviews) [15,16]. With a literature exceeding more than 1000 papers now, literally no reference cites a *reversible* technique delivering greater analgesia. Under certain circumstances, however, other techniques deliver equivalent analgesia, patient acceptability, or even fewer side effects. Patient-controlled narcotic delivery, for instance, achieves high marks for patient acceptability without the pruritus and urinary retention associated with spinal narcotics like morphine [17]. However, this pertains to short periods of use, as during postoperative pain therapy. The proper approach defines the pain syndrome, adequacy of prior analgesic therapy, and finally whether the patient is likely to respond to spinal narcotic prior to instituting therapy. Other considerations then surface in the decision to institute spinal narcotic analgesia. Should spinal narcotic be started early or late in the terminal course? Is the risk of a side effect or infection sufficient to preclude early intervention with spinal narcotic? What are the indications for specific methods of spinal narcotic delivery? Fortunately, since all the consequences of spinal narcotic trials are reversible, the patient can be tested with spinal narcotic bolus prior to placing a system for spinal narcotic delivery [18]. The likelihood of success or failure can be predicted to some extent, thus avoiding false hope and unnecessary procedures for these desperate patients.

Patients with intractable cancer pain are frequently said to constitute the most appropriate indication for chronic narcotics. This attitude was appropriate when intraspinal narcotic analgesia was a new, largely unproven technique. A more seasoned situation now exists, with substantial experience in many centers and some understanding of the situations in which spinal narcotics may fail to control cancer pain. In the main, failure is due to one of the five causes listed in table 6-2 [19]. This inevitably leads one to consider the pathophysiologic mechanisms (aside from

Table 6-2. Causes of spinal narcotic failure

---

1. Neurogenic or incident pain/deafferentation
2. Failure of delivery system/inadequate dose[a]
3. Tolerance/tachyphylaxis[a]
4. Obstructed CSF mechanics, i.e., epidural tumor
5. Emotional decompensation

---

[a] Note: Reverse side of inadequate dose is aggressive or uncontrolled disease. A rare cause of failure is hyperalgesia from concentrated morphine (see text).

misdiagnosis, psychoemotional decompensation, and failure of delivery systems) that result in pain unresponsive to spinal narcotic.

Though cancer progresses at different rates in individual patients, the pattern per se does not produce pain resistant to spinal narcotic. Similarly, some degree of tolerance to narcotic arises in all patients (older patients appear to manifest less tolerance in general) but this factor does not preclude successful narcotic analgesia. In contrast, certain syndromes are very resistant to narcotic analgesia irrespective of the route of delivery [20]. Thus, the spinal narcotic resistance of the syndrome is perhaps proportional to the extent to which a narcotic-resistant type of pain dominates a given pain complex [21]. For example, reflex sympathetic dystrophy, neurogenic pain, edematous swelling, ischemia, inflammation, bone destruction, and deafferentation may all be present in a patient with Pancoast syndrome and brachial plexopathy. However, narcotic resistance will vary tremendously by virtue of which components dominate and what personality composite underlies the syndrome.

Review of the spinal narcotic literature sheds little light on this particular issue. Unfortunately, in the cancer patients treated with spinal narcotics, the type of pain is not classified in such away that the comparative response to spinal narcotic can be judged. The singular exception is a report by Arner and Arner from Scandinavia [21]. The components and patterns of cancer pain are classified in this series of 55 patients treated with epidural morphine. On the basis of this preliminary approach, it appears that somatic and visceral pain, whether constant or intermittent in pattern, are reasonably controllable with epidural morphine. In contrast, cutaneous and nuerogenic pain were quite resistant. Several difficulties impeded both research and clinical application of this data. First, the comparability of patients as to prior narcotic and adjunctive analgesic exposure is limited and in any event difficult to arrange prospectively. Second, the predominance of a truly resistant component in these patients is unknown and again difficult to characterize prospectively. However, Chabal recently found no correlation between this type of classification and the ability to control cancer pain with spinal narcotic [22]. Dominance by a particular pain mechanism in either study is central to interpretation. More research will be required to resolve this issue. However, the concept as presented by Arner and Arner is valuable and instructive. Practically, one can determine the balance by simply assessing the response to an intrathecal narcotic bolus. One last point must be made: intrathecal and epidural narcotic may not be comparable since some degree of

Table 6-3. Spinal-narcotic-resistant types of pain (ascending magnitude)

1. Continuous somatic
2. Continuous visceral/intermittent somatic
3. Intermittent somatic
4. Cutaneous/RSD
5. Deafferentation
6. Neurogenic incident (i.e., radicular)
7. Pain with epidural tumor

supraspinal narcotic activation is sure to occur with the epidural approach [23]. Intrathecal doses of polar drugs like morphine are much less likely to do this, especially during continuous infusion rather than bolus delivery [24]. Thus, an intrathecal bolus is more likely to predict in isolation success with spinal opioid-receptor-mediated analgesia as opposed to some combination of spinal and supra-spinal influences.

Table 6-3 lists the components of pain in ascending order of resistance to spinal narcotic. Conceptually, this list is a composite of the author's impressions and other published work. The incidence of totally resistant pain syndromes is fairly low, probaly representing only about 5–15% of cases treated with spinal narcotics [25–31]. Of course, those treated with spinal narcotics tend to represent a composite of difficult-to-treat cancer patients or conventional narcotic therapeutic failures. To be fair, some are also patients treated by anesthesiologists with little experience with cancer pain therapy. Walsh reported that only about 2% of referrals to a collaborative multicenter cancer pain clinic trial in Denmark were candidates for spinal narcotic analgesia [25]. In their studies, 11% of these Danish pain patients developed serious resistance to spinal narcotics irrespective of the cause.

Before proceeding to a discussion of clinical approaches to the use of spinal narcotic agents, reference to some recent animal studies may shed some light on narcotic resistance associated with some pain syndromes. A variety of acute pain models have been employed to assess the spinal potency of analgesics, including cutaneous thermal tests such as tail flick and hot-plate tests and visceral stimulation of which the peritoneal irritant tests, such as acetic acid writhing in the rat, are representative. Yaksh, Schmauss, and colleagues have compared various classes of opioid-receptor agonists in these paradigms, demonstrating the following: 1) there are at least three opioid-receptor subclasses in the spinal cord that subserve analgesia, as demonstrated in the rat, monkey, and man; and 2) these three subclasses—mu, delta, and kappa opioid receptors—demonstrate a different hierarchy of potencies depending upon the type of pain-stimulus test [33–36]. With respect to cutaneous thermal and electrical stimulation versus visceral pain stimuli, mu receptors demonstrate activity in both models. Most strikingly, visceral pain was more responsive to kappa agonists while electrical thermal pain responded to delta agonists when the two were compared. This indicated for the first time that, at the spinal level at least, pain is modulated preferentially by different spinal receptors depending upon the source of stimulation. This further suggests that selective agonists will be needed to combat different types of pain.

Though morphine is the only opioid analgesic approved for spinal use, there is evidence that narcotics with affinity for several receptors indeed will have increased activity in some difficult-to-treat cases. Carl, Crawford, and colleagues reported an interesting preliminary series of patients, the majority of whom had cancer pain [30]. A smaller subset had nonmalignant pain. Both morphine and the partial mu agonist, buprenorphine, were used; the latter drug is interesting in that it has high lipid solubility, partial mu agonist activity, and some kappa-receptor affinity. The majority of cases initiated with either epidural morphine (83) or buprenorphine (51) were successfully controlled with the single agent used—61% and 72%, respectively. Those failing were crossed over to the other spinal drug. Buprenorphine controlled 46% of the cross-overs while only 32% of morphine-treated cross-overs succeeded. Buprenorphine-treated patients also had a lower incidence of side effects—20% versus 46% for morphine. This suggests that an alternative opioid agonist with kappa activity may add something over and above selective mu agonists. Unfortunately, no systematic neurotoxicology has been done on kappa agonists to facilitate FDA approval. A few clinical studies have evaluated the weaker agonist–antagonists, butorphanol and nalbuphine, in postoperative pain and labor [37,38]. They may have limited potenital, however, due to the greater relative potency of morphine and other narcotic agonists.

Anecdotal reports document the use of the delta-selective opioid agonist, DADL, to treat cancer pain and morphine tachyphylaxis [39,40]. Though generally successful, this peptide is not likely to become available soon [18]. At issue is whether and which patients with resistance to spinal morphine will respond to spinal delta agonists; a corollary question is whether clinical cross-tolerance will occur between mu- and delta-receptor agonists at the spinal level. We encountered a patient with neurogenic and deafferentation pain and advanced morphine tachyphylaxis who also demonstrated cross-tolerance to DADL [41]. Other potential options may emerge and are dealt with in a later section.

Certain syndromes are often associated with narcotic resistance, such as Pancoast-type brachial plexopathy. Resistance in this plexopathy is often due in part to the combined presence of neurogenic, reflex sympathetic, and deafferent type pain [20]. This situation may not completely respond to available spinal narcotics either. The possibility exists, however, that the greater apparent potency and duration of spinal narcotic analgesia may permit such cases to be adequately treated with spinal drug, alone or in partnership with adjunctive drugs, such that neuroablative or neurolytic procedures may be avoided [42]. Despite this alternative, other options, especially neurosurgery, will often be needed [18].

SPINAL AGONISTS FOR CANCER PAIN

Historically, cancer patients were the first patients treated with spinal narcotic. Wang and colleagues treated 10 pelvic cancer patients with 1/2 to 1 mg of intrathecal morphine, and compared the intensity and duration of analgesia to an

Table 6-4. Spinal agents for cancer pain

Agent	Route	Starting Dose (mg) bolus
Morphine[a]	E/I	5–10/0.3–1.0
Fentanyl	E	.050–2.0//0.1–0.3
Hydromorphone	E/I	1.0–2.5
Methadone	E	5–10
Buprenorphine	E	0.15–0.30
Bupivacaine[a]	E/I	15–75/hr//0.125/hr

[a] Note: These agents have been given by continuous infusion. Representative doses for bupivacaine infusion only are listed above. An adjustment to dosage based upon equivalent conversion from individual systemic narcotic intake is suggested in the text. Abbreviations: E = Epidural, I = Intrathecal.

intrathecal saline bolus [43]. The duration of pain relief exeeded 24 hours in some cases. Notably, striking placebo effects were also seen in some patients with saline. The potency of the clinical effects predicted by Yaksh and other early neuro-pharmacologists was confirmed [44]. Behar and Magora soon reported that this spinal analgesia extended to epidural narcotics in cancer pain and other settings [45]. Given the simplicity of the approach, the long history of narcotic use, development within a specialty long used to spinal cannulation, and the philosophical issues associated with cancer pain therapy, it is not surprising that extended use of spinal narcotics has flourished among anesthesiologists. A variety of spinal narcotics has now been used to treat cancer pain both acutely and chronically, although as noted earlier only morphine is approved for this purpose. The list shown in table 6-4 includes meperidine, hydromorphone, methadone, and buprenorphine, among others. Notably, only buprenorphine significantly demonstrates apparent activity at receptor sites besides the mu receptor. Clinical studies and some spinal neurotoxi-cology exist for the short duration and generally for lipophilic, synthetic 4-anilinopiperidines such as fentanyl, sufentanyl, and alfentanyl [46]. However, the short duration of activity has generally dissuaded most investigators from extended trials, since continuous infusion would appear to be the only logical alternative for delivery. Furthermore, their primary advantage—regional selectivity based on lipid solubility and thus lowered risk of respiratory depression—seems to be a nonissue. Respiratory depression and other CNS toxicity have rarely been reported in cancer patients, probably due to their history of prior narcotic exposure. Thus, for practical purposes, this review concentrates primarily on the use of morphine as a chronic spinal analgesic. Where appropriate, alternatives are stressed, along with the preferred route and delivery mode.

Morphine, used both as the sulfate in the USA and the chloride in Europe, has generally been effective in relatively low doses. The epidural route has been preferred to intrathecal delivery although systems exist to utilize both routes [18]. Few reports indicate the basis for establishing an effective dose schedule. In practice, most anesthesiologists will titrate the epidural dose with relative ease using percutaneous catheters or intermittent intrathecal boluses. Some guidelines are appropriate since this may not always be straightforward. Generally, we have converted the patient's daily systemic narcotic intake to I.M. morphine equivalents using the conversion tables developed by Houde and colleagues and popularized by Foley [47]. The starting epidural dose is then taken as 5–10% of daily systemic morphine equivalent with allowance for age, debility, prior narcotic exposure, and recent CNS depression. Similarly, the initial intrathecal dose is 1/2–1% of the systemic morphine equivalent dose per 24 hours [48]. Both are then given on a schedule based upon the duration of effective analgesia achieved with bolus dose. For example, the 65-year-old patient taking 200 mg/day I.M. morphine equivalents is started on a 10-mg epidural dose. A TID schedule is elected if the first dose gives good pain relief for 8–10 hours. When tachyphylaxis develops, dose frequency is increased first and dosage amount only later. We have used this approach successfully for over seven years to deduce starting doses irrespective of route and mode of delivery. Several considerations may influence dosage, including advanced age, infirmity, and prior narcotic exposure. In the presence of these factors, bolus techniques may expose the patient to greater risk of respiratory depression. In some cases, the enormity of terminal suffering precludes protracted trials to establish the perfect dose. A neurolytic block may be more appropriate in such situations. However, if practical, a short course of intrathecal morphine may decide the issue in favor of one particular approach.

Published trials with epidural and intrathecal morphine are difficult to interpret, but several investigators have accumulated significant series. Zenz and colleagues in West Germany found that percutaneous epidural morphine, and more recently buprenorphine, allowed satisfactory home care, in some cases exceeding a year [48,49]. Though an early report noted no significant tolerance development during the first 25 days of therapy, a subsequent report indicated that substantial increases were needed in some patients. This demonstrates tachyphylaxis at the opioid receptor. Subsequently, investigators from Denmark and Scandinavia have documented prolonged control of pain using a variety of narcotics, although morphine has been the principal agent [50,51]. Andersen and colleagues reported that the majority of patients are effectively controlled with epidural narcotic injections with the following positive results: home care is possible with the help of patient, family, local nurses, and personal physicians; acceptable but definite increases in spinal narcotic occurred with minimal difficulty from side effects; and finally, no cases of respiratory depression occurred despite phenomenal doses of epidural morphine in some cases.

Several other anecdotal reports testify to the efficacy of the technique [21,22,26,29,31,50,52–55]. Several qualifications must be made relative to most of these reports, however [1]. First, most of them do not classify the patients studied in such away that even minimal degrees of comparability exist within the groups studied; for example, type of tumor, site of pain, type or pattern of pain, pretherapeutic doses of analgesics, and adjunctive drugs are not controlled for. None of the studies to date have studied a control group, performed a cross-over, or made adjustments for changing baselines over time. Further, the use of measurement devices to assess pain and functional activity are missing in many cases. Lastly, few studies have linear controls for the impact of depression, psychological state, or cognitive integrity. Studies are ongoing in several centers to assess these issues. Hopefully this work will establish their proper context relative to conventional analgesic failure and more aggressive procedures for pain control. Until then, the tremendous acceptance by both patients and clinicians worldwide appears to support acceptable efficacy. Further justification is garnered from the fact that analgesia has been realized generally when conventional therapy failed. Perhaps failures are more notable than successes in deducing the limits of spinal narcotic therapy. In this regard, failure occurs for a variety of reasons, including several that have nothing to do with reduced response of the spinal opioid receptor. This area will be dealt with again in the section on Side Effects and Limitations.

TECHNIQUES FOR SPINAL NARCOTIC DELIVERY

A number of considerations relating to this methodology have been recently reviewed by this author and will only be highlighted [1,18]. In basic terms, the options for chronic spinal drug delivery are three: percutaneous catheters, subcutaneously implanted multiple injection ports, and permanently implanted infusion reservoirs. With the latter two options, either the epidural or intrathecal route may be selected. With continuous-delivery systems, either continuous fixed-rate flow pumps or programmable pumps with pacemaker-type controllability are available. Although interesting, the cost of programmable systems to date has been prohibitive without demonstrated efficacy over and above continuous-flow systems or the other options available [27]. Under certain circumstances, the greater complexity of implanted injection ports or infusion reservoirs may counterbalance the relative disadvantages of percutaneous systems and warrant the higher cost and occasional inconveniences of implanted systems. The potential factors influencing these decisions are listed in table 6-5. Some considerations overlap all three choices and will be addressed in the following subsections as questions.

Where should the spinal catheter be placed?

The choice hinges upon whether to use intrathecal or epidural drug delivery and at what vertebral level to insert the catheter and locate the catheter tip. The answer is integrally related to whether a percutaneous catheter is to be used. If the chronic percutaneous route is chosen, the risk of serious infection probably precludes chronic percutaneous techniques either because of short longevity, expenses of more elaborate systems, or other mitigating factors. Of those to be treated with implanted systems, no major differences in efficacy or complications have been shown between the epidural and intrathecal routes [56]. We base this decision primarily upon the following consideration: 1) some types of resistant pain may require combined use of local anesthetics and narcotics for optimum pain control, as a corollary; 2) local anesthetic therapy of pain above the diaphragm requires thoracic vertebral catheterization to establish regional block with the minimum volume of agent; and

Table 6-5. Factors influencing delivery system choice

	Percutaneous Catheter (tunnelled)	Port	Pump
1. Predicted survival	2 wks–2 mths	1 month	4 months
2. Local anesthetic capability	+ + +	+ + +	+
3. Support personnel requirements	+ +	+ + +	+
4. Technical difficulty	+	+ + +	+ + +
5. Expense	$200	$300–700	$1500–10,000
6. Intrathecal route feasability	No	Yes	Yes

ª Note: Relative magnitude in each category is scaled 0 (lowest magnitude) to + + + (significant/greatest magnitude). * Local anesthetics can be given via any system, however, as indicated in the text, this capability changes with level and site of catheter and other considerations.

3) chronic epidural cannulation leads to progressive reactive leptomeningeal fibrosis around catheters [24]. These factors would appear to stalemate decisions. In practice, however, when pain involves a substantial component of neurogenic pain or reflex sympathetic activity, we place an epidural catheter at a level to permit treatment with local anesthetic and then establish the delivery system in series with the optimal catheter placement.

The spinal activity of narcotics such as morphine is dependent on the proportion of the spinal dose reaching the CSF [44,57]. All dermatomal and metameric levels of pain afferents are thus treatable with a lumbar epidural or intrathecal catheter. The potential need for local anesthetic decides the ultimate epidural catheter location. In some cases, it is possible to fluoroscopically guide catheters rostrally from a lower insertion level. An alternate solution is to use double-lumen epidural catheters or two-port implanted injection ports. In the latter case, one port is used to access a lumbar epidural catheter placed for narcotics injection; the other port attaches to a thoracic epidural catheter, for example, for high thoracic local-anesthetic use.

Clearly, systems can be modeled to fit specific patient problems. By this same reasoning, implantable pumps should be chosen with an auxiliary injection port to permit bolus injections, CFS sampling if intrathecal in location, and diagnostic studies with local anesthetics or radiographic contrast dyes [18].

Fibrosis around epidural catheters may have many consequences. This leptomeningeal reaction may result in pain on injection, unpredictable spread of local anesthetic or narcotic solutions, reduced dural penetration of epidural drugs (particularly lipophobic agents like morphine) causing an apparent tachyphylaxis, and eventually obstruction or plugging of catheter lumens [19,58]. Rarely, spinal cord compression from pericatheter fibrosis has required surgical decompression [59]. During continuous infusion, these issues have seldom necessitated replacement of catheters. However, Crawford et al. [50] noted that pain on injection, inability to inject, and dislodgement of catheters led to catheter replacement 215 times in 105 patients treated with chronic epidural morphine. Looking into the future, it may not be necessary to employ the epidural route in order to use combined spinal narcotics and local anesthetics. Recent neurotoxicologic work in dogs at Rush–Presbyterian along with some preliminary results in man suggests that prolonged intrathecal bupivacaine delivery is both feasible and controllable [60]. This work may have substantial application for both short-term therapy of spinal narcotic tolerance and more chronic control of neurogenic and other resistant types of cancer pain.

Technical aspects of chronic spinal cannulation

The reliability and complication rate of chronic spinal delivery systems can be improved by several techniques to facilitate retention of spinal catheters and reduce infection risks. Both the type of catheter and the method of fixation deserve mention. Our own experience indicates that somewhat larger and heavier silastic catheters are easier to anchor, less likely to kink or obstruct, and are reasonably well tolerated by patients. Further, whether multiorificed or not, these conduits are less likely to cannulate epidural veins. The latter complication may not be detected, is easily ruled out at the time of implantation by injection of a water-soluble contrast agent during fluoroscopy, and is a rare cause of spinal narcotic resistance. We anchor both epidural and intrathecal catheters to the supraspinous ligament with a figure-eight 2-0 silk suture [19]. This necessitates that a small incision be made, of course. This incision is then utilized to pass a tunneling instrument to the flank or upper chest wall depending upon the vertebral level of catheter entry and sex of the patient. The percutaneous spinal catheter is then anchored again to the skin at the point of exit. Tunneling is important to reduce the risk of infection with chronic catheters much as with chronic hyperalimentation catheters.

Several aspects of chronic intrathecal cannulation require embellishment. Chronic dural leaks can be potentially ruinous. In addition to the risk of spinal headache, infection and subdural hematoma may result. Also it is possible that the resultant CSF pseudomeningocele may become large enough to dilute the narcotic injected while increasing the absorptive surface. This is another rare reason for spinal narcotic resistance. The previously described technique for anchoring the catheter in the supraspinous ligament has nearly eliminated our incidence of troublesome CSF leakage. Alternatively, the intrathecal catheter must be placed through a minilaminotomy with intramuscular tunneling of the exiting catheter as first described by Onofrio [61]. Though no data exist to the contrary, it must be surmised that the absolute risks of serious infection in the immunosuppressed cancer patient are increased with repetitive percutaneous intrathecal injections of narcotic agents through implanted ports. Thus most clinicians still prefer to place chronic epidural catheters when the system involves an implanted injection port.

Side effects and limitations

Fortunately, the side effects of intraspinal narcotic analgesia are less limiting in cancer patients than in acute postoperative use. This discrepancy is thought to occur primarily from prior narcotic exposure and presumed partial opioid tolerance [16,44]. Table 6-6 lists the common side effects associated with spinal narcotic use. Pruritus, nausea, emesis, and urinary retention do occur in the cancer patient treated

Table 6-6. Side effects of spinal opioids

---

1. Nausea
2. Pruritus
3. Urinary retention
4. Edema
5. Dysphoria/depression
6. Respiratory depression

---

with spinal narcotic. The impact, however, is less pronounced, and patients tend to become tolerant of these side effects rapidly. Rare patients are so sensitive to morphine, experiencing persistent nausea or emesis, that an alternative must be found. Hydromorphone has been the first alternative in our clinic for such cases. Alternatively, buprenorphine, meperidine, or sufentanyl may be substituted with appropriate attention to relative potencies and kinetics. Though most are availale in preservative-free preparations, none have been exhaustively studied for neurotoxicity or approved by the FDA. In some cases concern for the patient's suffering overrides these issues. In general, meperidine is not a good candidate for long-term use due to the potential for side effects from its metabolite, normeperidine [62]. The applicability of this concern to spinal use of meperidine is yet undefined. Notably, meperidine has substantial local anesthetic activity, making it somewhat effective as a spinal anesthetic [63]. Inadvertent intrathecal injection of volumes and doses meant for epidural use could therefore be dangerous. However, this local-anesthetic side effect of meperidine could be used to advantage to achieve the same effect as dilute intrathecal local anesthetic. This area deserves further exploration.

Respiratory depression, the potential scourage of postoperative analgesia with spinal narcotic use, is virtually unreported in the cancer patient treated with epidural approaches or continuous intraspinal infusion. Rare cases are known wherein patients received large intrathecal boluses [64]. However, striking doses have been injected in some cases of resistant pain, approaching 150 mg per day in one case reported by Greenberg [65]. Clearly some sense must be applied to both choice of starting dose (as outlined earlier) and rate of dosage escalation. Fortunately, this and most side effects of spinal narcotics are reversible with a narcotic antagonist such as naloxone. This fact has caused us to make available naloxone kits and educational training in their use of families of our cancer pain patients treated as outpatients. Family members may give naloxone in emergenies or after consultation as a potential antidote to build up of sedative- or coma-producing levels of spinal narcotic and systemic analgesic. We are especially concerned about the potential risks of spinal narcotic and dopamine-antagonist tranquilizer coadministration, a situation that occasionally arises in deafferented patients. This combination has been associated with respiratory depression in postoperative patients. Pain is a strong aversive to respiratory depression. However, when unrelieved pain is suddenly controlled or eliminated by neurolysis or cordotomy in a patient on high-dose spinal narcotic,

Table 6-7. Complications of implanted spinal drug delivery systems

1. Infection
2. Leakage of septums/catheters
3. System failure (block catheter, pump stoppage)
4. System migration
5. CSF leak/headache
6. Skin erosion over septum/system surfaces
7. Pain/discomfort from surrounding tissues, i.e. rib pain, wound discomfort, etc.

there may be some risk of respiratory depression, as has been reported with high-dose systemic narcotics [66].

Many of the potential complications of chronic spinal narcotic therapy relate primarily to the risks of the systems used to deliver drugs. A partial list of these complications is shown in table 6-7. Most of these problems do not require reiteration. The risks of spinal infection are not precisely known with most of these systems. Estimates range between 7% in Zenz series of epidural catheters to 2% in a recent report by Chabel [22,48]. Zenz encountered two cases of meningitis among 105 patients so treated. None proved fatal. In contrast, reports of infection with totally implanted systems are as yet rare, although if comparable to hip prosthesis, a 1–2% incidence should prevail. The incidence of implantable pump failure is likely about 1% with continuous flow systems [19]. The potential to develop septum leaks exists with all implantable systems. This usually requires in excess of 1000 punctures with most available systems. This magnitude will only be reached with injection ports, making this issue less of a concern with infusion pumps. Nevertheless, small huber-tip needles should be used for injecting all implantable systems, coupled with meticulous skin preparation and aseptic technique.

TOLERANCE, ABSTINENCE SYNDROMES, AND NEUROTOXICITY

Tolerance and narcotic abstinence syndromes are problems unique to chronic as opposed to acute spinal narcotic use. Theoretically, patients treated previously with high-dose systemic narcotic may develop narcotic withdrawal syndromes when spinal narcotic therapy is instituted without systemic narcotic weaning. Reports of this problem have surfaced occasionally [67]. This presumably occurs because the systemic levels of narcotic achieved during spinal opioid use are not sufficient to prevent withdrawal at tolerant supraspinal opioid receptors.

The differential diagnosis of tolerance or tachyphylaxis and methods to overcome this problem are listed in table 6-8. Technical difficulties with delivery systems must be ruled out first. A variety of psychological and pathophysiologic events may confuse the issue. Attempts must be made to delineate components of the pain process that are amenable to simple adjunctive therapy. Local anesthetic blocks for cancer-associated RSD, antiepileptics for deafferentation, and steroid administration to reduce bone pain may all help individual patients. Similarly, some patients will require specific antidepressant therapy to treat psychological depression. Often progressive spinal narcotic escalation is appropriate during phases of rapid disease progression. However, how much is too much? Clearly, when high doses or impaired clearance of narcotics yield excessive sedation, confusion, or other CNS toxicities, other approaches must be sought. In our experience, little further analgesia is gained from escalating spinal morphine doses beyond 250–300 mg/day epidurally or 20–30 mg/day intrathecally. If these simple alternatives are exhausted and the situation precludes a neurodestructive alternative, we will attempt to treat the patient's pain with regional local anesthetics, as for example by the epidural route. During this holiday from pain, the spinal and systemic narcotics are withdrawn and the patient is detoxified. Often therapy can be reinstituted with morphine or another spinal alternative for a time. This procedure is rarely completely satisfactory. It does have the advantage of forestalling a crisis until the patient can regroup coping mechanisms and the physician can come to a firm diagnosis and new treatment strategy. The patient may now be able to accept another alternative, or time can be gained to initiate new chemotherapy, radiation, or spinal analgesic trials.

Several circumstances invariably seem to foreshadow failure of spinal narcotic therapy [56]. The development of spinal or epidural tumor compression will not be overcome by spinal narcotic. The narcotic may not penetrate to the spinal cord area compressed. Further CSF obstruction will prevent ascendance of narcotic beyond the block [24]. Relatedly, the multiplicative interaction between descending inhibitory pathways activated by morphine, and intrinsic interneuronal inhibitory systems in the dorsal horn is functionally severed by compression [68]. Thus no attempt should be made to treat patients with spinal narcotic without ascertaining the integrity of the spinal CSF column. An important corollary follows. Look for epidural tumor encroachment or epidural infection in patients unrelieved of their pain during spinal narcotic therapy.

A peculiar situation has been identified by Yaksh while investigating the potential neurotoxicity of high concentrations of morphine preparatory to any FDA approval. Yaksh found that concentrated morphine solutions injected intrathecally generated a painful withdrawal reaction in rats [69]. This phenomenon had also previously been seen by Wolfe [70] in rats with intrathecal morphine glucuronides. Yaksh and colleagues have presented evidence that this morphine hyperalgesia occurs via a spinal glycinergic inhibition somewhat akin to the action of strychnine [69]. This side effect seems to occur with morphine concentrations greater than 25 mg/ml and has been described anecdotally in the clinical setting. Here is the ultimate paradox: the agent given to relieve pain may indeed cause further pain. On the brighter side, this phenomenon has not been observed at least in animals with intraspinal injection of anilino–piperidine type synthetic narcotics in Yaksh's studies.

FUTURE TRENDS

The future remains quite bright for developing an array of selective spinal agonists that antinociceptively inhibit pain at the dorsal horn level in the spinal cord. Since both intrinsic spinal inhibitory circuits and descending pathways converge at least within the dorsal horn, both are theoretically amenable to attack by new agents. Further, combinations of agents with both receptor activity and local anesthetic action should find use for difficult pain syndromes. The possibility exists therefore to avoid procedures that permanently disrupt the neuraxis in order to control pain. Continuous intrathecal local anesthetic delivery has been mentioned. In our laboratory we have concentrated on activating the terminal synapses of the descending bulbspinal inhibitory pathways through the use of intrathecal and epidural alpha$_2$ adrenergic agonists, such as clonidine. There is substantial evidence in both animal and man that clonidine is a potent spinal analgesic [41,71,72]. It is also analgesic when spinal narcotic tolerance or resistant pain exists. Other inhibitory systems are currently under study including somatostatin and GABAergic receptor agonists [73,74]. Further, the search is on for acceptable spinal opioid agonists with selective activity at kappa or delta receptors for the potentially selective action they may possess against pain syndromes [34,39]. Kappa agonists appear not to produce urinary retention and have less risk potential for depressing respiratory drive [75]. Other potential advantages may also be found for kappa and delta agonists.

In summary, the pain-specialist anesthesiologist can now improve the analgesic outlook for many cancer pain patients by the judicious use of spinal narcotic techniques. Spinal narcotic analgesia may be adapted dynamically to changing requirements, thus permitting a functionally better quality of life while perhaps forestalling or avoiding the need for neurodestructive procedures in some cases.

REFERENCES

1. Coombs DW (1985): New approaches to chronic pain therapy. Semin Anesthes 4:287–299.
2. Foley K (1985): The treatment of cancer pain. N Eng J Med 313:84–95.
3. Bonica JJ (1980): Cancer pain. In: Bonica JJ (ed), Pain. New York: Raven Press, pp 335–362.
4. Bond MR (1979): Psychological and emotional aspects of cancer pain. In: Proceedings of International Symposium on Pain of Advanced Cancer. Bonica JJ, Ventafridda V (eds), Advances in Pain Research and Therapy, vol 2. New York: Raven Press, pp 81–88.
5. Sternbach RA (1974): Pain Patients: Traits and Treatment. New York: Academic Press.
6. Derogatis LR, Morrow G, Fetting S, et al. (1983): The prevalence of psychiatric disorders among cancer patients. JAMA 250:751–757.
7. Twycross RG, Lack SA (1983): Symptom Control in Far Advanced Cancer: Pain Relief. London: Pitman Books Ltd, pp 167–189.
8. Foley KM (1982): The practical use of narcotic analgesics. In: Reidenberg MM (ed), The Medical Clinics of North America. Philadelphia: W.B. Saunders, pp 1091–1104.
9. Nahata MC, Miser AW, Miser JS, Reuning RH (1984): Analgesic plasma concentrations of morphine in children with terminal malignancy receiving a continuous subcutaneous infusion of morphine sulfate to control severe pain. Pain 18:109.
10. Portenoy RK (1985): Continuous intravenous infusions of narcotics. In: Management of Cancer Pain: Syllabus of the Postgraduate Course Memorial Sloan-Kettering Cancer Center, November 14–16, 1985. New York: Memorial Sloan-Kettering Cancer Center, pp 205–214.
11. Baumann TJ, Batenhorst RL, Graves DA, Foster TS, Bennett RL (1986): Patient-controlled analgesia in the terminally ill cancer patient. Drug Intell Clin Pharm 20:297–301.
12. Terenius L (1985): Families of opioid peptides and classes of opioid receptors. In: Fields HL, Dubner R, Cervero F (eds), Advances in Pain Research and Therapy, vol 9. New York: Raven Press, pp 463–477.
13. Coombs DW, Saunders RL, Gaylor M, et al. (1982): Epidural narcotic infusion reservoir: Implantation technique and efficacy. Anesthesiology 56:469–473.
14. Advokat C (1985): Evidence of place conditioning after chronic intrathecal morphine in rats. Pharmacol Biochem & Behav 22:271–277.

15. Yaksh TL, Noueihed R (1985): The physiology and pharmacology of spinal opiates. Ann Rev Pharmacol Toxicol 25:433–462.
16. Cousins MJ, Mather LE (1984): Intrathecal and epidural administration of opiates. Anesthesiology 61:276–310.
17. Rosenberg PH, Heino A, Scheinin B (1984): Comparison of intramuscular analgesia, intercostal block, epidural morphine, and on-demand-i.v. fentanyl in the control of pain after upper abdominal surgery, Acta Anaesthesiol Scand 28:603–607.
18. Coombs DW (1986): Management of chronic pain by epidural and intrathecal opioids: Newer drugs and delivery systems. In: Sjostrad UH, Rawal N, (eds), Regional opioids in anesthesiology and pain management. International Anesthesiol Clin 24:59–74.
19. Coombs DW (1985): Continuous Spinal Morphine Analgesia for Relief of Cancer Pain, lst edition. Cambridge, MA: Shea Bros, pp 1–29.
20. Kanner RM, Martini N, Foley KM (1982): Incidence of pain and other clinical manifestations of superior pulmonary sulcus (Pancoast) tumors. In: Bonica JJ, Ventafridda V, Pagni CA (eds), Advances in Pain Research and Therapy, vol 4. New York: Raven Press, pp 27–39.
21. Arner S, Arner B (1985): Differential effects of epidural morphine in the treatment of cancer related pain. Acta Anaesthesiol Scand 29:32–36.
22. Chabal C, Buckley FP (1987): Long-term epidural narcotic analgesia in the treatment of cancer pain (Abst.). Reg Anesthes 12:22–23.
23. Chauven M, Samii K, Sherman J, et al. (1981): Plasma concentrations of morphine after IM, epidural, and intrathecal administration of low doses of morphine. Br J Anaesth 53:911–913.
24. Coombs DW, Fratkin JD, Meier F, et al. (1985): Neuropathologic lesions and CSF morphine concentrations during chronic continuous intraspinal morphine infusion: A clinical and post mortem study, Pain 22:337–351.
25. Eriksen J, Andersen HB (1984): Pain treatment on long term basis using extradural opiates. Pain (Suppl 2) 19:S335.
26. Wang J (1985): Intrathecal morphine for intractable pain secondary to cancer of pelvic organs: Clinical note. Pain 21:99–102.
27. Penn RD, Paice JA, Gottschalk W, Ivankovich A (1984): Cancer pain relief using chronic morphine infusion. J Neurosurg 61:302–306.
28. Krames ES, Gershow J, Glassberg A, Kenefick T, Lyons A, Taylor P, Wilkie D (1985): Continuous infusion of spinally administered narcotics for the relief of pain due to malignant disorders. Cancer 56:696–702.
29. Rico RC, Hobika GH, Avellanosa AM, Trudnowski RJ, Rempel J, West CR (1982): Use of intrathecal and epidural morphine for pain relief in patients with malignant disease: A preliminary report. Journal of Medicine 13:223–231.
30. Carl P, Crawford ME, Ravlo O, Bach V (1986): Long-term treatment with epidural opioids. Anaesthesia 41:32–38.
31. Yablonski-Peretz T, Klin B, Beilen Y, Warner E, Baron S, Olshwang D, Catane R (1985): Continuous epidural narcotic analgesia for intractable pain due to malignancy. J Surg Oncology 29:8–10.
32. Walsh TD (1984): Oral morphine in chronic cancer pain. Pain 18:1–11.
33. Yaksh TL (1983): In vivo studies on spinal opiate receptor systems mediating antinociception: I. mu and delta receptor profiles in the primate. J of Pharmacol and Exp Therap 226:303–316.
34. Schmauss C, Yaksh TL (1983): In vivo studies on spinal opiate receptor systems mediating antinociception: II. Pharmacological profiles suggesting a differential association of mu, delta, and kappa receptors with visceral chemical and cutaneous thermal stimuli in the rat. J Pharmacol and Exp Therap 228:1–12.
35. Przewlocki R, Stala L, Greczec M, Shearman GT, Przewlocki B, Herz A (1983): Analgesic effects of mu-, delta-, and kappa-opiate receptor agonists and, in particular, dynorphin at the spinal level. Life Sci 33:649–652.
36. Porreca F, Mosberg HI, Omnas JR, Burks TF, Cowan A, (1987): Supraspinal and spinal potency of selective opioid agonists in the mouse writhing test. J Pharmacol Exp Therap 240:890–894.
37. Naulty JS (1985): Intraspinal narcotics. In: Obstetric Analgesia and Anaesthesiology I. Ostheimer GW (ed), Clinics in Anesthesiology. East Sussex, Great Britain: W.B. Saunders Co., pp 145–156.
38. Mok MS, Lippman M, Wang JJ, et al. (1984): Efficacy of epidural nalbuphine in postoperative pain control. Anesthesiology 61:A187.
39. Onofrio BM, Yaksh TL (1983): Intrathecal delta-receptor ligand produces analgesia in man. Lancet 1:1386.

40. Krames ES, Wilkie DJ, Gershow J (1986): Intrathecal D-Ala^2-D-Leu^5-enkephalin (DADL) restores analgesia in a patient analgetically tolerant to intrathecal morphine sulfate. Pain 24:205–209.
41. Coombs DW, Saunders RL, Lachance D, Savage S, Ragnarsson TS, Jensen LE (1985): Intrathecal morphine tolerance: Use of intrathecal clonidine, DADL, and intraventricular morphine. Anesthesiology 62:358–363.
42. Coombs DW, Saunders RL, Maurer LH, Hensen LE (1987): Continuous intraspinal narcotics for cancer pain in cervicothoracic dermatomes. Reg Anesthes 12:26–27.
43. Wang JK, Nauss LE, Thomas JE (1979): Pain relief by intrathecally applied morphine in man. Anesthesiology 50:149–151.
44. Yaksh TL (1981): Spinal opiate analgesia: Characteristics and principles of action. Pain 11:293–346.
45. Behar M, Olshwang D, Magora F, Davidson JT (1979): Epidural morphine in treatment of pain. Lancet 1:527–529.
46. Yaksh TL, Noueihed RY, Durant PAC (1986): Studies of the pharmacology and pathology of intrathecally administered 4-anilinopiperidine analogues and morphine in the rat and cat. Anesthesiology 64:54–66.
47. Houde RW (1979): Systemic analgesics and related drugs. In: Bonica JJ, Ventafridda V (eds), Advances in Pain Research and Therapy, vol 2. New York: Raven Press, pp 263–273.
48. Zenz M, Shappler-Scheele B, Neuhans R, Piepenbrock S, Hilfrich J (1981): Long-term peridural morphine analgesia in cancer pain. Lancet 1:91.
49. Zenz M ( ): Epidural opiates for the treatment of cancer pain. In: Zimmerman M, Drugs P, Wagner G (eds), Recent Results in Cancer Research vol 89. Heidelberg: Springer Verlag, pp 107–115.
50. Crawford ME, Andersen HB, Augustenborg G, et al. (1983): Pain treatment on out-patient basis utilizing extradural opiates: A Danish multicentre study comprising 105 patients. Pain 16:41–46.
51. Eriksen J, Andersen HB (1984): Pain treatment on long term basis using extradural opiates. Pain (Suppl 2), S335.
52. Findler G, Olshwang D, Hadani M (1982): Continuous epidural morphine treatment for intractable pain in terminal cancer patients. Pain 14:311–315.
53. Dagi TF, Chilton J, Caputy A, Won D (1986): Long-term, intermittent percutaneous administration of epidural and intrathecal morphine for pain of malignant origin. The American Surgeon 52:155–158.
54. Howard RP, Milne LA, Williams NE (1981): Epidural morphine in terminal care. Anaesthesia 36:51–53.
55. Poletti CE, Cohen AM, Todd DP, Ojemann RG, Sweet WH, Zervas NT (1981): Cancer pain relieved by long-term epidural morphine with permanent indwelling systems for self-administration. J. Neurosurg 55:581–584.
56. Coombs DW, Maurer LH, Saunders RL, Jensen LE (1984): Outcomes and complications of continuous intraspinal narcotic analgesia for cancer pain control. J Clin Oncol 2:1414–1420.
57. Nordberg G (1984): Pharmacokinetic aspects of spinal morphine analgesia. Acta Anaesth Scand (Suppl 79) 28:1–38.
58. Coombs DW, Fratkin J (1987): Neurotoxicology of chronic spinal analgesics (editorial). *Anesthesiology* (in press).
59. Rodan BA, Cohen FL, Bean WJ, Martyak SN (1985): Fibrous mass complicating epidural morphine infusion. Neurosurgery 16:68–70.
60. Kroin JS, McCarthy RJ, Penn RD, Kerns JM, Ivankovich AD (1987): The effect of chronic subarachnoid bupivacaine infusion in dogs. Anesthesiology (in press).
61. Onofrio BM, Yaksh TL, Arnold PG (1981): Continuous low-dose intrathecal morphine administration in the treatment of chronic pain of malignant origin. Mayo Clin Proc 56:516–520.
62. Kaiko RF, Foley KM, Grabinski PY, Heidrich G, Rogers AG, Inturrisi CE, Reidenberg MM (1983): Central nervous system excitatory effects of meperidine in cancer patients. Ann Neurol 13:180–185.
63. Famewo CE, Naguib M (1985): Spinal anaesthesia with meperidine as the sole agent. Can Anaesth Soc J 32:533–537.
64. Cobb CA, French BN, Smith KA (1984): Intrathecal morphine for pelvic and sacral pain caused by cancer. Surg Neurol 22:63–68.
65. Greenberg HS, Taren J, Ensminger WD, Doan K (1982): Benefit from and tolerance to continuous intrathecal infusion of morphine for intractable cancer pain. J Neurosurg 57:360–364.
66. Hanks GW (1981): Unexpected complications of successful nerve block: Morphine induced respiratory depression following removal of severe pain. Anaesthesia 36:37–39.

67. Tung AS, Jenicela R, Winter PM (1980): Opiate withdrawal syndrome following intrathecal administration of morphine. Anesthesiology 53:340.
68. Yeung JC, Rudy TA (1980): Multiplicative interaction between narcotic agonisms expressed at spinal and supraspinal sites of antinociceptive action as revealed by concurrent intrathecal and intra-cerebroventricular injections of morphine. J Pharmacol Exp Therap 215:633–642.
69. Yaksh TL, Harty GJ, Onofrio BM (1986): High doses of spinal morphine produce a nonopiate receptor mediate hyperesthesia: Clinical and theoretic implications. Anesthesiology 64:590–597.
70. Wolfe CJ (1981): Intrathecal high dose morphine produces hyperalgesia in the rat. Brain Res 209:491–495.
71. Yaksh TL, Reddy SVR (1981): Studies in the primate on the analgesic effects associated with intrathecal actions of opiate, alpha adrenergic agonists, and baclofen. Anesthesiology 54:451–467.
72. Coombs DW, Saunders R, Gaylor M, Lachance P, Jensen L (1984): Clinical trial of intrathecal clonidine for cancer (Abstr). Reg Anes 9:28.
73. Chrubasik J, Meynadier J, Blond S, Scherpereel P, Ackerman E, Weinstock M, Bonath K, Cramer H, Wunsch E (1984): Lancet 2:1208–1209.
74. Penn RD, Kroin KS (1985): Continuous intrathecal baclofen for severe spasticity. Lancet 2:125–127.
75. Dray A, Metsch R (1984): Opioid receptor subtypes involved in the central inhibition of urinary bladder motility. Eur J Pharmacol 104:47–53.

7. APPLICATION OF ELECTRICAL CURRENT TO THE CENTRAL NERVOUS SYSTEM FOR RELIEF OF PAIN

SANFORD J. LARSON, M.D., PH.D.

Twenty years ago, Shealy and associates reported that application of electrical current to the dorsal columns of human patients was associated with relief of pain below the level at which the currents were applied [14]. These observations were confirmed by subsequent reports [10,15]. The selection of the dorsal columns for electrode placement was based upon the gate theory proposed by Melczak and Wall [8], who suggested that impulses conducted over large afferent fibers activated cells of the substantia gelatinosa that in turn affected small-fiber input by presynaptic inhibition. Subsequently, the theory was modified to include activation of descending fibers from higher levels [9]. Additional hypotheses that proposed to account for relief of pain associated with application of current to the nervous system have included release of opiatelike substances such as endorphin [12].

As experience with application of current to the dorsal columns accumulated, it became apparent that regardless of the validity of the gate theory, it could not account for the relief of pain experienced by many patients [4,6]. As the intensity of the applied currents was increased, each patient described paresthesias that correspondingly increased in intensity. While many reported relief of pain, in others the paresthesias became intolerable before relief of pain was achieved. In some patients, decreased perception of joint rotation, pain, and touch, combined with hyperactive deep reflexes, pathological reflexes, and ankle clonus developed before pain relief was reported. These neurological changes always disappeared after the currents were turned off. When a sensory level developed, it was always at the level at which the electrodes were applied, although paresthesias were experienced several segments

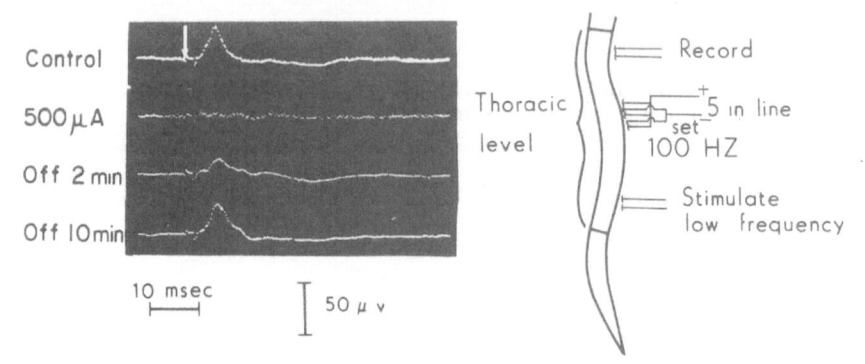

Figure 7-1. Recordings of cord-to-cord evoked potentials before, during, and after current application to five in-line electrodes on the dorsal surface of the cord. The stimulating and recording electrodes are separated by the five in-line current electrodes. Barbiturate anesthesia. Analysis time is 62 msec. stimulus at arrow. Response obliterated with 500 μA peak pulse current applied to five-electrode set. Recovery at approximately 10 minutes after 100 Hz current is off. (From Larson St. et al. [4].)

higher. Relief of pain was reported only in the area of analgesia, but persisted in the area of paresthesia above the level. Since the large fibers bifurcate as they enter the spinal cord, and the descending limb proceeds several levels caudad, it is not surprising that paresthesias were experienced at levels above those at which the currents were applied. The relief of pain only in the analgesic segments suggested that the applied currents were blocking afferent transmission in the fiber pathways serving pain perception, and that pain relief was not secondary to inhibition of small fibers by large-fiber activity. To test this hypothesis, experiments were conducted in monkeys in whom electrodes of alternate polarity were chronically implanted on the spinal cord [4]. Application of current through these electrodes blocked transmission in those portions of the axon immediately beneath the electrodes (figures 7-1, 7-2) while responses secondary to stimulation and recording using electrodes either both above or both below the level of current applications were unaffected (figure 7-3). Although the currents blocked axonal transmission, these effects were reversible and histological examination did not demonstrate any neuronal damage even with long-term application of current.

Although most patients obtained good initial relief of pain with application of current to the dorsal columns, this effect progressively diminished in those with extended survival times, although paresthesias continued without change. Since pain relief appeared to depend upon block of transmission in the spinothalamic tracts, these changes could be explained by thickening of the dura and arachnoid beneath the electrode moving the electrodes farther away from the spinal cord with a consequent decrease in current density in the spinothalamic tract.

To determine the effect of application of current to the anterior portion of the spinal cord, electrode sets were implanted on the anterior and on the posterior

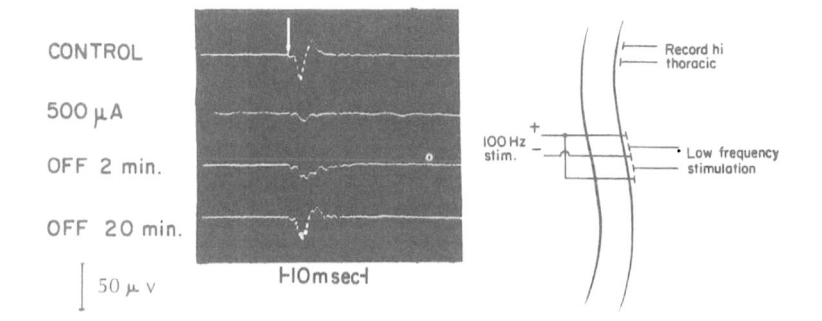

Figure 7-2. Potentials recorded from bipolar electrodes on the dorsal aspect of the spinal cord (upper thoracic) above the five-electrode set evoked by stimulation through electrodes 2 and 4 of the five inline array before, during, and after application of current at 100 Hz through electrodes 1, 3, and 5. Barbiturate anesthesia. Analysis time is 31 msec, stimulus at arrow. Response is reduced with 500 μA pulse current applied to electrodes 1, 3, and 5. Recovery approximately 20 minutes after 100 Hz current is off. (From Larson SJ et al. [4].)

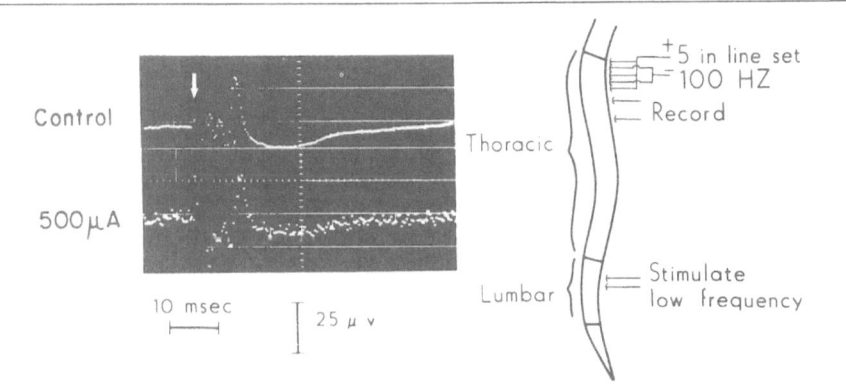

Figure 7-3. Recordings of the potentials evoked from the cauda equina to the lower thoracic spinal cord. Stimulating and recording bipolar electrodes are both below the five in-line current electrodes. The responses are unaffected by the applied currents. Noise on the lower trace is due to applied currents. Analysis time is 62 msec, stimulus at arrow. (From Larson SJ et al. [4].)

surfaces of the thoracic portion of the monkey spinal cord [6]. Other electrodes were chronically implanted in specific and nonspecific afferent pathways. Stimulation of the contralateral peripheral nerve evoked responses of short latency in sensorimotor cortex and nucleus ventralis posterior lateralis of the thalamus. The responses recorded from the intralaminar nuclei had a longer latency and could be obtained with both ipsilateral and contralateral stimulation. When currents were applied at 100 per second through the posterior electrode sets, the responses recorded from sensorimotor cortex, VPL, and the medial lemniscus were abolished while with corresponding levels of current the responses recorded from the intralaminar nuclei

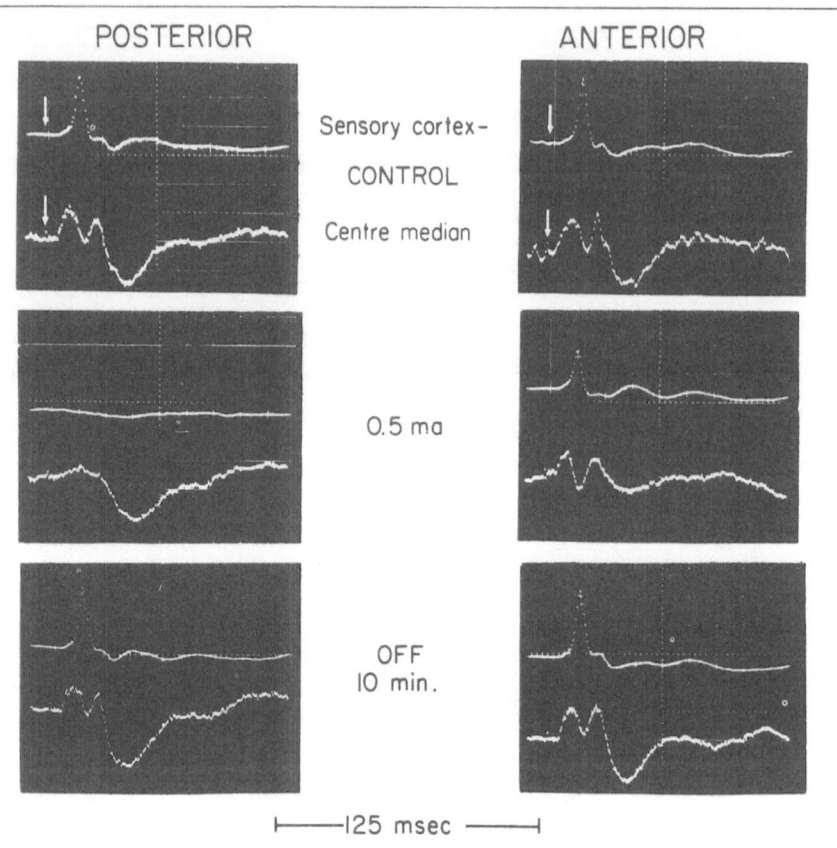

Figure 7-4. Responses recorded from monkey sensory cortex and nucleus centre median secondary to peripheral stimulation. Early deflection in CM response reflects activity in medial lemniscus. Recordings in left- and right-hand columns indicate effects of application of current at 100 Hz to posterior and anterior electrode sets, respectively. Arrow indicates shock artifact. (From Larson SJ et al. [5].)

were unaffected. On the other hand, when currents were applied at 100 per second to the anterior electrode sets, the responses to peripheral stimulation recorded from the intralaminar nuclei were abolished while the responses recorded from the electrodes in the specific somatosensory pathways were much less affected (figure 7-4). Consequently, it appeared that application of currents to the anterior surface of the spinal cord would more effectively block conduction in the spinothalamic pathways than would currents applied through the posterior electrode sets.

As a result of these experimental observations, similar electrode sets were implanted in patients with intractable pain secondary to metastatic cancer [6]. Each electrode set had its own receiver so that currents could be applied independently to either the anterior or to the posterior surfaces or to both simultaneously (figure 7-5).

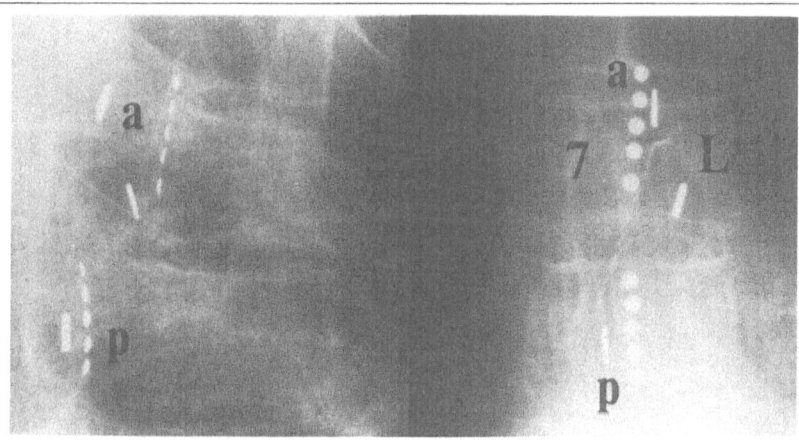

Figure 7-5. Lateral (left) and anteroposterior (right) spine films showing T6, T7, T8. Anterior electrode sets (a) are at T7, the posterior sets (p) at T8. (From Larson SJ et al. [5].)

When currents were applied to the anterior surface of the spinal cord, the patients did not experience paresthesia but did report relief of pain below the level of current application with development of sensory level for pain to approximately that at which the electrodes had been placed. The somatosensory evoked potential amplitude was unaffected (figure 7-6). Application of current through the posterior electrodes again produced paresthesias with reduction in amplitude of somatosensory evoked potentials (figure 7-7). In some patients, the amount of current applied to the anterior surface of the spinal cord to produce relief of pain and analgesia also produced painful muscle contraction in the distribution of the nerve roots at the level at which currents were applied. This phenomenon was particularly evident when the patients had pain in the sacral dermatomes, probably because it was necessary to deliver larger currents to the cord to achieve an appropriate current density in the peripherally located sacral spinothalamic fibers. To increase the amount of current that could be applied, rhizotomy at two levels was performed bilaterally. In some instances, a combination of anterior and posterior current application provided satisfactory relief without segmental root driving. Blocking of spinothalamic pathways also appeared to be more effective when two sets of electrodes were implanted anteriorly, one on each side of the midline [6].

Because the experimental and clinical observations suggested that when transmission in the spinothalamic tract is affected by currents applied through electrodes on the dorsal columns, the current density in the dorsal columns must necessarily be substantially higher than in the anterior quadrants. This accounts for the difficulty encountered in relieving pain in the lower lumbar and in the sacral segments, since paresthesias may become severe before an effective current density is achieved in the more lateral portions of the spinothalamic tract. Although application of current

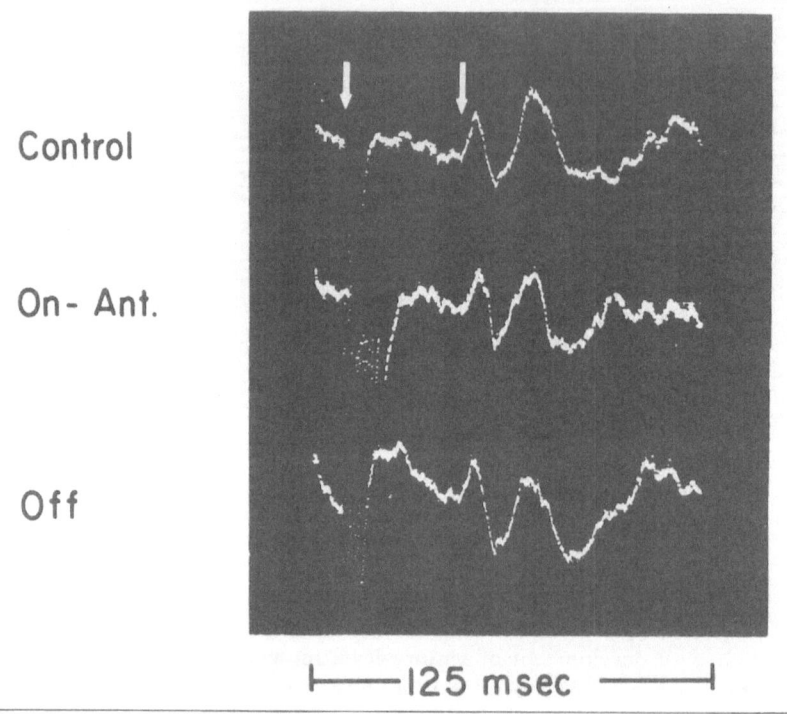

Control

On- Ant.

Off

├────125 msec ────┤

Figure 7-6. Potentials evoked by stimulation of contralateral peroneal nerve before (top), during (middle), and after (lower) application of sufficient 100 Hz current to anterior electrode set to produce analgesia and pain relief. First arrow indicates shock artifact; second arrow, onset of evoked potential waveform. (From Larson SJ et al. [5].)

through anteriorly placed electrodes provides analgesia and pain relief without paresthesias, discomfort associated with activation of anterior roots frequently limited the amount of current that could be applied.

In an effort to define the most effective electrode configuration, current density measurements were made in monkey and human cadaver spinal cord specimens with currents applied through various electrode configurations [16]. With currents applied either through anterior or posterior electrode systems, the current density was greatest in those portions of the spinal cord immediately beneath the electrodes, decreasing with distance from the electrode (figure 7-8). Although with the anterior electrode system, current densities were greater in the anterior qudrants than in the dorsal columns, nevertheless with each system the lateral-most portions of the spinothalamic tract had a very low current density. When currents were passed through the spinal cord from negative anterior electrodes to positive posterior electrodes, the highest current densities were found in the mid-sagittal plane near the electrodes, decreasing with distance lateral to the center of the cord. When electrodes of this type were implanted at the C2–C3 level in a patient with intractable pain in

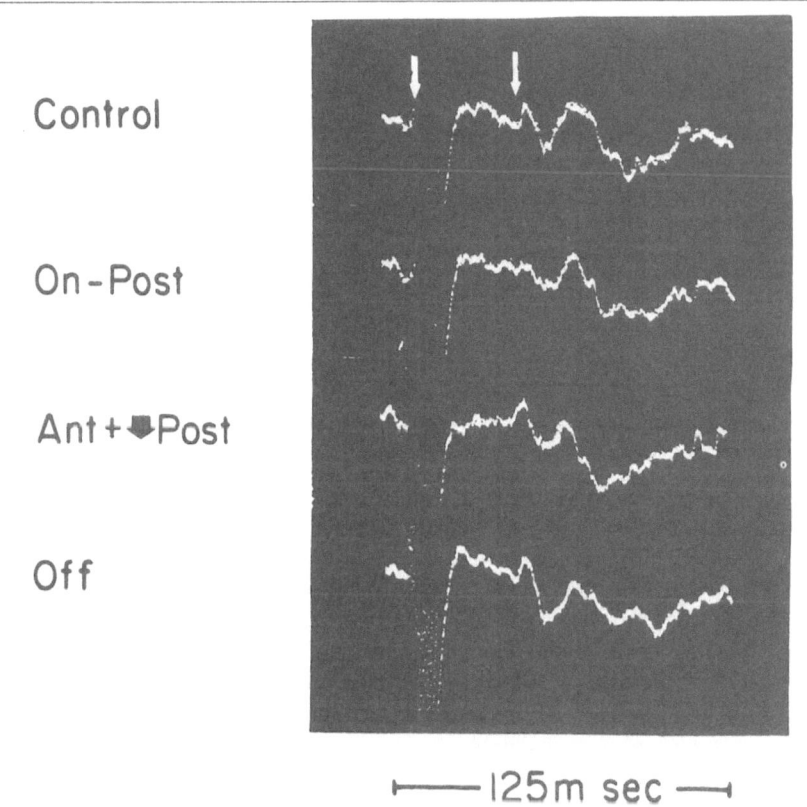

Figure 7-7. Potentials evoked by peroneal nerve stimulation in same patient as figure 7-5. Top recording is control, second was made after application of 100 Hz current to posterior electrodes, third was made after 100 Hz current was applied to anterior electrodes and reduced at posterior set, and fourth was made after currents were turned off. First arrow indicates shock artifact and second arrow indicates beginning of evoked potential waveform. (From Larson ST et al. [5].)

the left upper limb secondary to apical carcinoma of the lung, application of current was followed by analgesia between C3 and T8 with relief of pain [6]. Perception of touch and joint rotation were unaffected and somatosensory potentials evoked by transcutaneous stimulation of the median nerves were not affected. When the applied currents were increased beyond this point, tremulous movements appeared in the left hand but voluntary movement was not impaired. Currents applied through these electrodes appeared to affect the spinothalamic fibers from the cervical and upper thoracic dorsal horn neurons, producing dissociated sensory loss.

Although application of current to the spinal cord can effectively relieve pain in the thoracic and abdominal segments, lasting relief was not consistently achieved for perineal pain. Currents applied through the upper cervical spinal cord from negative anterior to positive posterior electrodes produced dissociated sensory loss in the

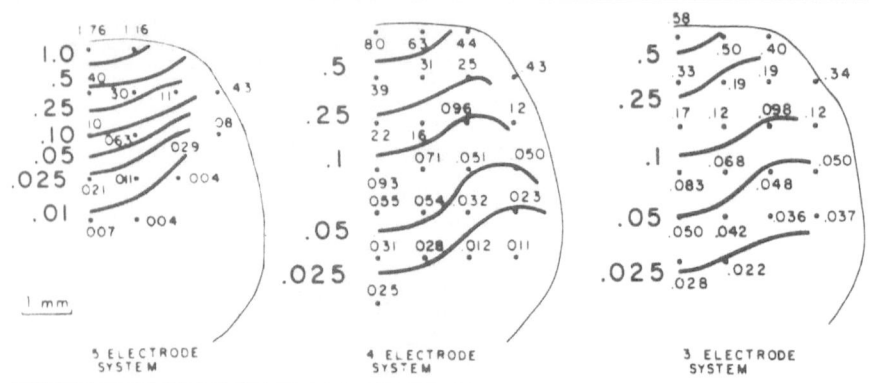

Figure 7-8. Current density in cadaver cord (mA/cm²). Current density readings have been superimposed over a tracing of an enlarged photograph of a cross section of a cadaver cord used in the experiments. Current flow is essentially orthogonal to the cross section at points shown. Boldface lines were hand drawn between the points showing actual measurements. (From Swiontek TJ et al. [16].)

upper limbs without driving of motor roots, probably because this portion of the cord is wide enough to permit a sufficient current density in the mid-sagittal region without reaching levels in the more lateral portions great enough to drive the anterior horn cells. However, when this configuration was applied in the thoracic portion of the cord, motor root driving became a problem. Therefore, the anterior posterior configuration is not suitable for use in the terminal portion of the cord where the electrodes must be applied if perineal pain is to be relieved, since rhizotomy here would impose an unacceptable neurological deficit. Consequently, except for pain in the upper limbs, thoracoabdominal areas, and perhaps proximal portions of the lower limbs, application of current to the spinal cord has not been useful over the long term. The type of pain that is best treated by interruption of afferent pathways is that located in the lower limbs and perineum and is unfortunately not effectively relieved with application of current to the spinal cord. Therefore, the use of spinal implants for relief of pain associated with metastatic disease is limited. Since electrodes placed directly on the cord frequently do not provide an effective intramedullary current density, it is clear that percutaneously placed epidural sets will be even less effective.

Application of current through electrodes with the tip located in the periaqueductal gray has been reported to relieve pain without paresthesias other than a sensation of warmth [11,12]. Perception of pain was sometimes reduced in patients with cancer during application of current and for variable periods thereafter. Although good relief of pain was achieved, survival time following implant was less than three months. One of the hypotheses advanced to account for the relief of pain secondary to delivery of current in the region of the periaqueductal gray was activation of an endogenous opiate system with release of opiatelike peptides [12]. However, lesions in this area produce contralateral loss of pain and temperature related to interruption of the spinothalamic tract, and it is therefore possible that currents applied through electrodes in this region block transmission in the spinothalamic tracts. Although application of currents through electrodes in the periaqueductal region offers an alternative to ablative procedures in patients with intractable head and neck pain, these operations are infrequently required because of improved methods for treatment of head and neck cancer.

Currents have also been applied through electrodes located in the posterior limb of the internal capsule and in various thalamic nuclei in patients with intractable pain other than of neoplastic origin [1,2,3]. The effect was always on the side contralateral to the electrodes. Although various hypotheses have been proposed to account for the relief of pain associated with current application in these regions, all of the observations can be accounted for by block of afferent pathways subserving pain perception. Although theoretically this type of implant could be used in patients with cancer, application would appear limited to those with head and neck pain. For pain on both sides of the body, bilateral implants would be necessary [1,3].

Because experiments conducted to determine the mechanism of electroanesthesia had demonstrated that diffuse transcranial currents produced unresponsiveness by blocking cerebral cortical activity [13], it appeared likely that localized application of current could produce focal interference with cortical function. If this were true, then application of current through electrodes placed on the cortex could be expected to produce loss of sensory perception in the underlying areas with relief of pain. Such a procedure would be expected to have less potential complications than might be associated with introduction of depth electrodes into the brain stem, diencephalon, or internal capsule. Experiments conducted in monkeys demonstrated that because of the large amplitude of the currents applied to the cortex, recordings could not be made during application [5]. However, the reduction in amplitude of the cortical response to stimulation of the contralateral peripheral nerve persisted after the cortical currents were discontinued, and consequently could be demonstrated. The responses recorded from VPL and from spinal cord secondary to low-frequency application of current to the cortex were reduced during concomitant high-frequency application of current (figure 7-9A,B). Since these observations suggested that localized application of current to the cortex could block cortical function, electrodes were chronically implanted in a patient with intractable pain from head and neck cancer (figure 7-10), who had received maximal surgical and radiation therapy and was requiring increasing amounts of narcotic analgesics without adequate relief of pain. He was unwilling to have an ablative procedure such as thalamotomy, tractotomy, or rhizotomy. The electrodes were placed over face and arm areas that had been identified by evoked potential recording and then were connected to a subcutaneous receiver. Application of current through the implanted electrodes at 100 per second produced decreased perception of all modalities in the face, neck, and upper limb contralateral to the electrodes. The reduction in amplitude of evoked potential was proportional to the intensity of the current applied (figure 7-11) and was similar to the effects produced by topical application of local anesthetic to the cortex during surgery (figure 7-12A,B). The pain was

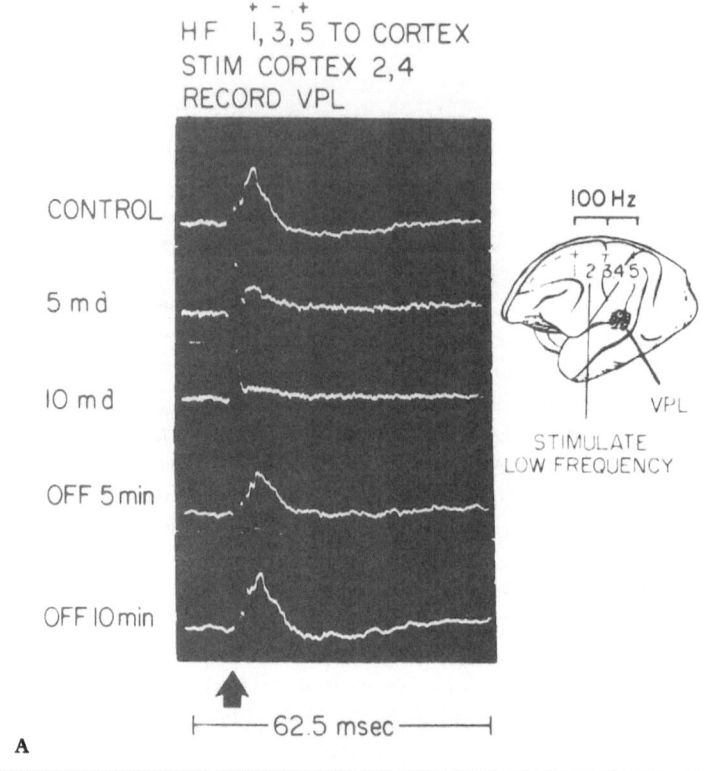

Figure 7-9A. Responses recorded from VPL evoked by low-frequency pulses applied through electrodes 2 and 4, before, during, and after application of current at 100/second through electrodes 1, 3, 5.

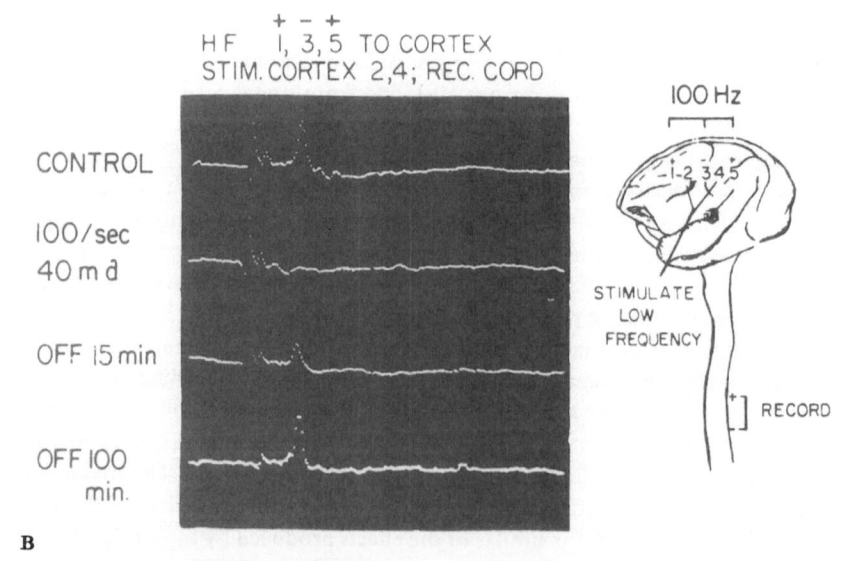

Figure 7-9B. Responses recorded from spinal cord under conditions similar to figure 7-9A.

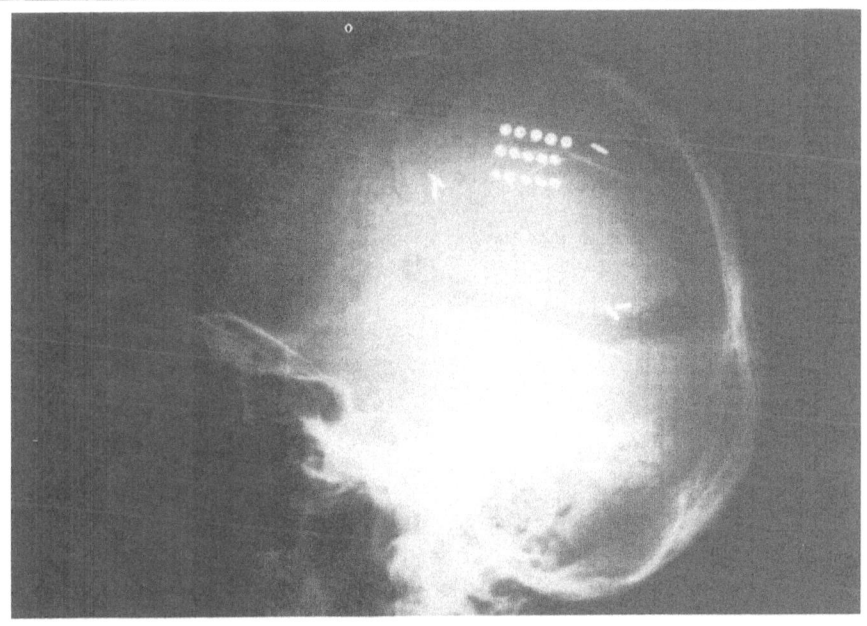

Figure 7-10. Electrodes chronically implanted over hand and face cortex as identified by evoked potential recordings.

effectively relieved during application of current and although perception of pain and evoked potential amplitude recovered within five minutes after the currents were turned off, relief of pain persisted for somewhat longer periods. The patient had been placed on anticonvulsants prior to application of current and did not develop generalized seizures. Nevertheless, if the amplitude of the current was increased too rapidly, focal facial seizures developed contralateral to the cortex stimulated. Although the possibility of neuronal damage secondary to current application exists, in this patient histological examination of the cerebral cortex using stains for degenerating myelin and standard stains for cell bodies did not demonstrate any evidence of neuronal injury connected with the currents, which were applied extensively over a period of two months [7]. Although the results of application of current to the cortex is interesting, this technique has limited applications, and its role appears limited to that of an alternative to cortical resection.

The relief of pain associated with application of electrical current to the central nervous system appears related to reversible conduction block in neurons subserving the perception of pain. Although effective in many patients, particularly in the earlier stages of illness, late results have been less satisfactory. As the disease progresses, pain breaks through, apparently because the conduction block secondary to application of current is less effective than actual interruption of the fibers of the spinothalamic tracts. Even with tractotomy, pain may recur in the final stages,

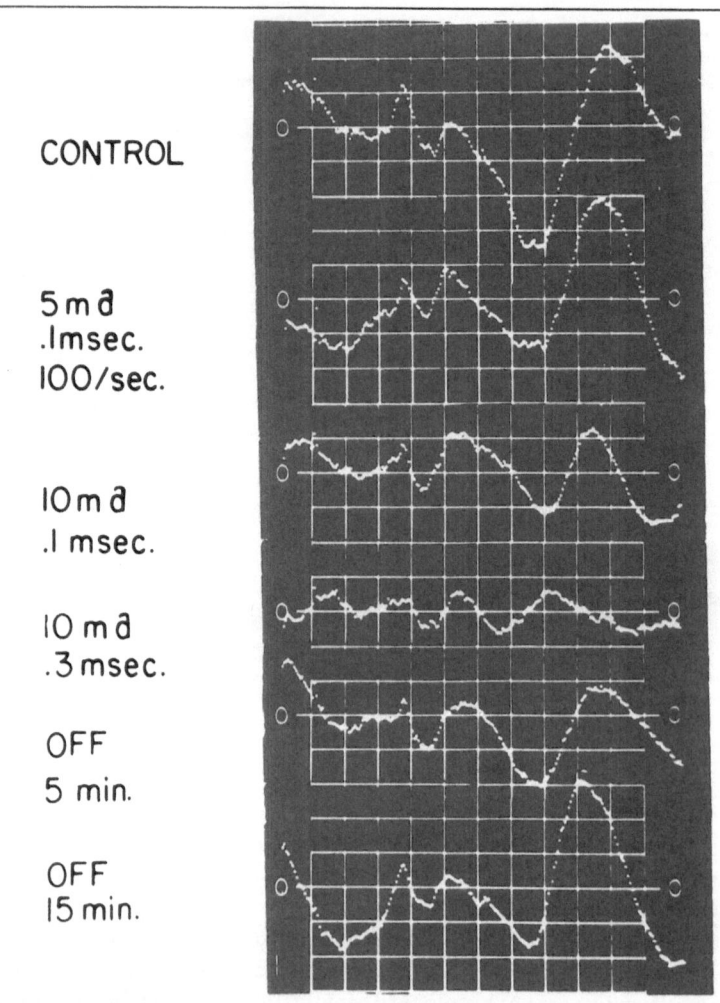

CONTROL

5 m ∂
.Imsec.
100/sec.

10 m ∂
.I msec.

10 m ∂
.3 msec.

OFF
5 min.

OFF
15 min.

Figure 7-11. Potential evoked by stimulation of a digital nerve recorded from scalp electrodes before and immediately after transcutaneous application of current to electrodes implanted over sensory motor cortex.

probably because neither reversible nor irreversible conduction block deals with the affective aspects of cancer pain.

REFERENCES

1. Adams JE, Hosobuchi Y, Fields HL (1974): Stimulation of internal capsule for relief of chronic pain. J Neurosurg 41:740–744.
2. Fields HL, Adams JE (1974): Pain after cortical injury relieved by electrical stimulation of the internal capsule. Brain 97:169–178.

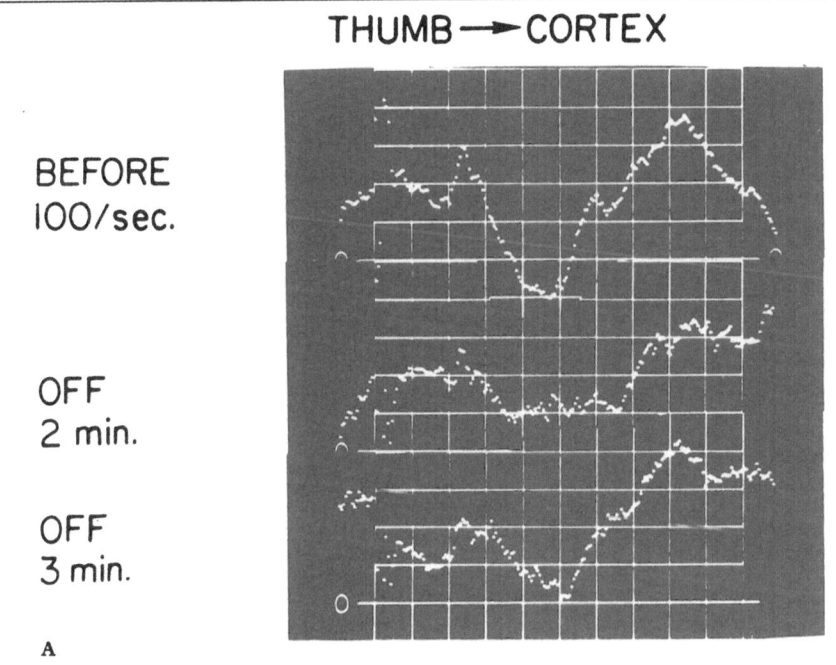

Figure 12A. Response evoked by stimulation of digital nerve of the thumb before and after application of current to sensory motor cortex through the implanted electrodes.

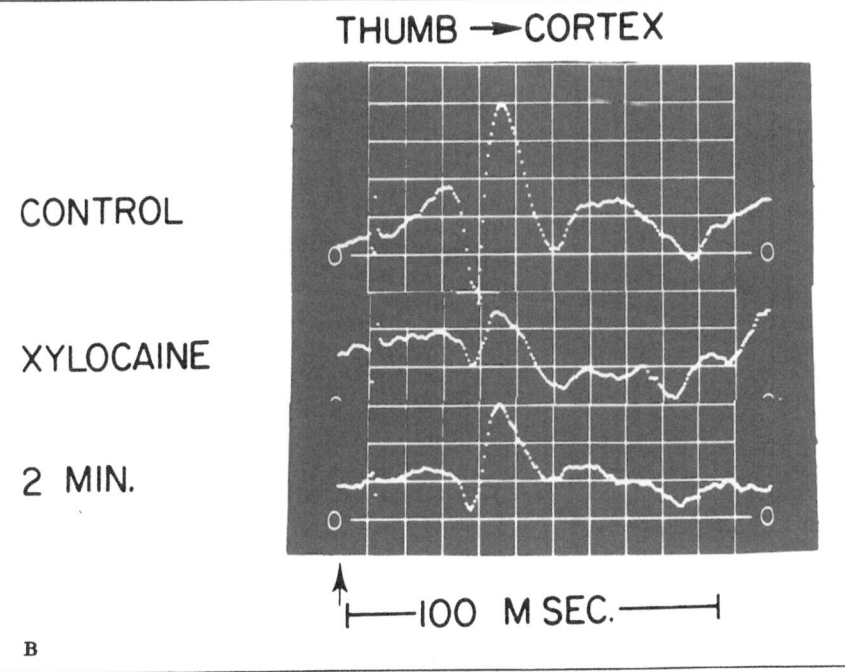

Figure 7-12B. Intraoperative recording of response similar to 12A before and after application of local anesthetic agent to the thumb area of sensory motor cortex.

3. Hosobuchi Y, Adams JE, Rutkin B (1975): Chronic thalamic and internal capsule stimulation for the control of central pain. Surg Neurol 4:91–92.
4. Larson SJ, Sances A Jr, Riegel DH, Meyer GA, Dallmann DE, Swiontek T (1974): Neurophysiological effects of dorsal column stimulation in man and monkey. J Neurosurg 41:217–223.
5. Larson SJ, Sances A Jr, Swiontek TJ (1974): Electronic block of sensory motor cortex in monkey and man. Proc of the Neuroelectric Society Ann Mtg, New Orleans, LA, Nov 20–23, p 55.
6. Larson SJ, Sances A Jr, Cusick JF, Meyer GA, Swiontek T (1975): A comparison between anterior and posterior spinal implant systems. Surg Neurol 4(1):180–186.
7. Larson SJ, Sances A Jr, Cusick JF, Myklebust J, Millar EA, Boehmer R, Hemmy DC, Ackmann JJ, Swiontek TJ (1976): Cerebellar implant studies. IEEE Trans BME 23:307–312.
8. Melzack R, Wall PD (1965): Pain mechanism: a new theory. Science 150:971–979.
9. Melzack R, Wall P (1970): Psychophysiology of pain. Int Anesthesiol Clin 8:3–34.
10. Nashold B, Friedman H (1972): Dorsal column stimulation for control of pain. J Neurosurg 36:590–597.
11. Richardson DE, Akil H (1977): Pain reduction by electrical brain stimulation in màn. Part 1: Acute administration in periaqueductal and periventricular sites. J Neurosurg 47:178–183.
12. Richardson DE, Akil H (1977): Pain reduction by electrical brain stimulation in man. Part 2: Chronic self-administration in the periventricular gray matter. J Neurosurg 47:184–194.
13. Sances A Jr, Larson SJ (1975): Electroanesthesia: Biomedical and Biophysical Studies. New York: Academic Press.
14. Shealy CN, Mortimer JT, Reswick JB (1967): Electrical inhibition of pain by stimulation of the dorsal columns: Preliminary clinical report. Anesth Analg Curr Res 46:489–491.
15. Shealy CN, Mortimer JT, Hagfors NR (1970): Dorsal column electroanalgesia. J Neurosurg 32:560–564.
16. Swiontek TJ, Sances A Jr, Larson SJ, Ackmann JJ, Cusick JF, Meyer GA, Millar EA (1976): Spinal cord implant studies. IEEE Trans BME 23(4):307–312.

8. NEUROLYTIC BLOCKS FOR CANCER PAIN

THERESA FERRER-BRECHNER, M.D.

Neurolytic blocks have been used to relieve cancer pain for more than 50 years, and yet fair to good results have remained at the 50–60% range [1]. There exists a need to redefine the role of neurolytic blocks in patients with cancer pain, given the advent of intrathecal and epidural morphine [2] and given the fact that advances in cancer therapy have succeeded significantly in prolonging the life expectancy of patients with cancer [3]. Recent studies have increased awareness with regard to the prevalence and severity of cancer pain, thus behooving us to take a closer look at the efficacy of neurolytic blocks.

Unfortunately, it is difficult to assess the realistic efficacy of neurolytic blocks, firstly because no standardized method of assessing treatment outcome has been utilized, and secondly because no comparison has been made with other pain-relieving methods currently available for controlling pain in cancer patients until demise.

At present, we still have a poor understanding of the indications, appropriate timing, and limitations of chemical neurolysis. Although it may provide prompt relief in some types of cancer pain, its long-term effect is questionable [4]. To understand fully the role of chemical neurolysis in cancer pain, we need to look at its proper place in the overall armamentarium of physical modalities available in a multidisciplinary setting [5,6]. This review will, therefore, look at the indications, types, and limitations of neurolytic blocks as they apply to the overall management of cancer pain.

Table 8-1. Substances commonly used for chemical neurolysis

Substance	Site Injected
Cryoanalgesia ($-60°C$)	Peripheral nerves [7]
Hypertonic saline	Intrathecal [8]
Chlorocresal	Intrathecal [9]
Ammonium sulfate (10%)	Peripheral nerve [10]
Phenol	
10% in 10% glycerol	Epidural [11]
	Sympathetic ganglia [12]
5–6% in 100% glycerol	Intrathecal [13]
Alcohol	
50%	Celiac [14]
100%	Intrathecal [15]

NEUROLYTIC AGENTS

Various substances have been applied to peripheral nerves, plexuses, and the intrathecal and epidural space. The types and concentration of these substances are dependent on the site of injection (table 8-1).

Cryoanalgesia is a new method of providing prolonged neural blockade. It involves freezing a peripheral nerve to $-60°C$ for one to two minutes and is particularly helpful in peripheral neuromas resulting from amputations and in facet arthalgia. The advantage of freezing is the reduced chance of inducing neuralgia, because the myelin sheath is preserved and normal regeneration of the nerve occurs. With injection of neurolytic agents, the myelin sheath is destroyed permanently, so that abnormal nerve regeneration can occur, inducing neuralgia several months later.

Intrathecal injection of hypertonic saline initially was advocated to block primarily the small C nociceptive fibers without affecting the sensory, motor and autonomic fibers [16]. Cerebrospinal fluid is withdrawn and replaced with 0.9% saline at 2–4°C up to a volume of 40–50cc [8]. The injection causes severe pain so that general anesthesia may be necessary. Complications can be severe, e.g., pulmonary edema, tachycardia, premature ventricular contractions [17], paralysis and paresthesia [18], and even death [19]. Pain relief is usually of short duration.

Ammonium sulfate, chloride or hydroxide, pitcher plant distillates, were thought to produce neural degeneration in 10% concentration or more. The effect is nonselective according to type of nerve fiber affected if injected peripherally in animals [20]. Intrathecal injection of ammonium salts has been done in human begins [21]. Complications consisted of nausea, vomiting, and headache, and if high doses were used, 30% of the patients had paresthesias and burning sensation lasting 2–14 days.

Phenol and alcohol are perhaps the more commonly used neurolytic agents in present times. Differences between these two agents are important for us to understand, especially when we are utilizing them for intrathecal use as seen in table 8-2.

Table 8-2. Phenol vs. alcohol for intrathecal neurolysis

	Phenol	Alcohol
Concentration	4–6%	100%
Diluent	Absolute glycerol	None
Baricity	Hyperbaric	Hypobaric
Pain on injection	-0-	+ + +
Site of action	Paravertebral somatic nerve	Dorsal root as it leaves spinal cord
Onset of action	15–20 minutes	Immediate
Position of patient	Lateral position flexed with target area in most dependent position and 45° tilt back	Prone position with target area in most superior position

For the novice anesthesiologist, it is best for intrathecal purposes to utilize phenol rather than alcohol, since phenol allows some margin for error in positioning. Phenol, upon contact with the somatic nerves, induces an immediate warm sensation projected to the dermatomal distribution of the nerves being bathed by phenol. However, neurolysis does not commence until 10–15 minutes later, thus providing the opportunity to reposition the patient if the warm sensation is not along the intended dermatomes. In contrast, alcohol initiates neurolysis immediately upon contact, thus disallowing any error in positioning. In addition, alcohol causes pain on injection. This may cause patient movement and inaccuracy of the block.

For epidural injection of phenol, ideal for pain in the chest wall and abdominal wall, a 10% solution of 10% glycerol is ideal [11]. Predictive block with 1% Lidocaine is done to determine the volume of 10% phenol necessary for neurolysis. It is important to allow an interim period of four to five hours between the local anesthetic and phenol injection to prevent the still unabsorbed Lidocaine from acting as a vehicle in spreading the phenol in more dermatomes than expected.

Pathological findings following alcohol and phenol injections have been studied in animal models as well as in post mortem examination in humans. When 95% alcohol is injected to a peripheral nerve, all fibers (sympathetic, sensory, and motor) are destroyed. In concentrations below 80%, the effects on motor fibers are reported to be variable. Injection of 60–80% alcohol into the sciatic nerve of pigs, rabbits, and cats resulted in prolonged paralysis, the duration of paralysis being unrelated to the concentration above 60% alcohol. Recovery from paralysis was not related to the pathologic evidence of nerve degeneration or regeneration [22]. In most studies, the period of time for motor-function recovery did not consistently correlate with the concentration of alcohol; 48% and 95% alcohol caused the same duration of paralysis in animals [23].

CRITERIA FOR NEUROLYTIC BLOCKS

The decision to proceed with neurolysis should occur only after thorough evaluation of physiologic, cognitive, and functional indications [24]. Physiologically, it is important to establish the pathophysiology of the pain syndrome, even if this requires repetition of radiologic diagnostic tests. The extent of the disease influences the decision to proceed with neurolysis. The extent of involvement should be localized enough for safe neurolytic block. For example, extension of a metastatic lesion to the lumbosacral plexus in a patient with intact bladder and bowel sphincter control would preclude the injection of a neurolytic substance into the plexus because of the high probability of sphincter and motor loss.

Another physiologic criterion to consider is the responsiveness of the tumor to chemotherapy and radiation therapy. Certain tumors provoking pain may dramatically diminish in size with the application of radiation therapy. Therefore, if chemotherapy or radiation therapy is applicable, enough time must be allowed before a neurolytic block is done for pain control. The presence of any coagulopathy or any active tumor at the site of infection precludes the use of neurolytic blocks.

Cognitive criteria to be satisfied in order to proceed with neurolysis include the ability of the patient and the family to understand the procedure and the risk–benefit ratio of the procedure. The procedure must be acceptable not only to the patient but also to the family. Report of pain intensity changes during diagnostic nerve blocking should parallel the physiologic changes that occur with local-anesthetic blocking. If the patient continues to experience pain despite a local-anesthetic block covering the dermatomal levels of pain, one should not proceed with neurolysis.

Functional criteria include weighing the benefit of the block against probable loss of function that may be associated with neurolysis. For example, the motor loss that can occur with intrathecal neurolysis of lumbar somatic nerves may not be acceptable to a patient who is still ambulatory.

To understand more clearly the appropriateness of neurolytic block in the overall management of cancer pain, one has to place in context the various modalities available for cancer pain control. The neurolytic blocks not only are indicated for specific conditions, but also need to be appropriately timed. Noninvasive, less risky therapy should be utilized first before proceeding to the more risky neurolytic blocks [25]. A decision tree is proposed to help clarify the appropriate indication and timing of neurolytic blocks as they relate to other existing modalities (Figure 8-1).

CHOICE OF NEUROLYTIC BLOCK

In this section, we will try to identify the neurolytic nerve blocks indicated according to the pathophysiology and dermatomal distribution of pain. This list is by no means complete.

Table 8-3 outlines the choice of diagnostic and therapeutic nerve block according to the pathophysiology of pain, i.e., whether pain is the nociceptive or deafferentation type in nature. Nociceptive pain results from noxious stimuli from bone, tissue, or viscera without evidence of neural damage. Examples are those pains arising from bone, visceral, or tissue metastasis. Patients with such pain usually have rapidly progressive disease, and have a shortened life expectancy. Neurolytic blocks are indicated in this group of patients for rapid pain relief. In contrast, deafferentation pain usually arises from partial to complete neural damage stemming from

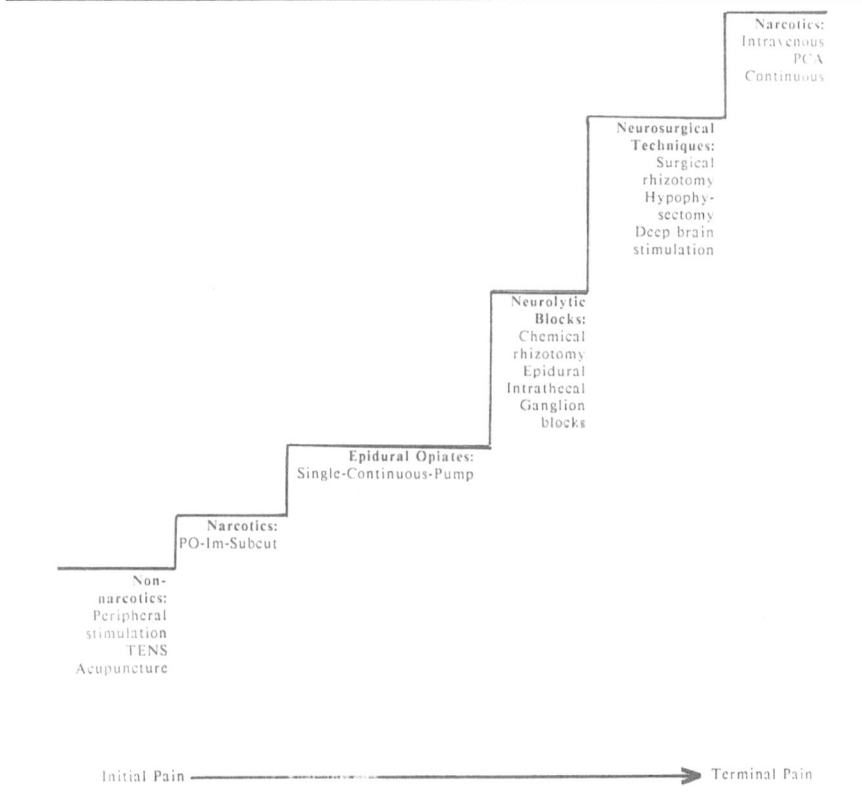

Figure 8-1. Ladder of physical modalities currently available for cancer pain management from early phase to terminal stages. The procedures become more invasive as the ladder escalates.

oncologic treatments. Examples are pains associated with postmastectomy, post-thoracotomy, postherpetic neuralgia or postchemotherapy neuropathy. Patients with this type of pain already have partial to complete denervation, and further denervation by neurolytic agents will aggravate deafferentation pain several months later. Unless life expectancy is three months or less, further denervation for patients with deafferentation pain is not indicated. Therefore, deafferentation with neurolytic blocks is indicated primarily for nociceptive pain, but not for deafferentation pain.

LIMITATIONS OF NEUROLYTIC BLOCKS

The factors that may limit success of neurolytic blocks are precision of needle location, predictability of success with prior local anesthetic blocking, and under-standing the pain-experience changes that occur with neurolytic block. Our colleagues and the referring physicians usually have a myth that neurolytic blocks are permanent, and therefore the recurrence of pain is considered a failure, even though such recurrence merely reflects the limited duration of the neurolytic agent.

Table 8-3. Choice of neuroablative procedures for cancer pain

	Nociceptive Pain	Deafferentation Pain
Face and oral cavity	Block of trigeminal ganglion and its branches	Upper and middle cervical ganglion block
Neck	Cervical plexus block: C_{2-3-4} somatic nerve block	Upper and middle cervical ganglion block
Shoulder and upper extremities	Cervical epidural or intrathecal block C_2-T_1	Stellate ganglion block
Chest wall	Intercostal nerve block or thoracic epidural T_1-T_8	Thoracic epidural T_2-T_8
Abdominal wall	Intercostal nerve block T_8-T_{12}	Thoracic epidural T_8-T_{12}
Abdominal viscera	Celiac plexus block	Celiac plexus block
Pelvic/perineum		
absent bladder/bowel function	Intrathecal phenol	Intrathecal phenol
intact bladder/bowel function	Epidural morphine	Epidural morphine
Lower extremities	Intrathecal phenol (L_1-L_5) or percutaneous chordotomy	Lumbar sympathetic block

Precision of needle placement

When small amounts of neurolytic agents are needed to block a specific somatic nerve, precision of needle location is of paramount importance. In a previous study, fluoroscopic guidance seems mandatory for paravertebral somatic nerve blocks, celiac plexus block, and sacral root blocks because of the high incidence of needle displacement even when suggested standard external landmarks are used [26].

With celiac plexus block, fluoroscope guidance is necessary to ensure location of needle tip anterior to T_{12} and L_1 (figure 8-2A). Injection of a small amount of air (figure 2B) or contrast media can ensure the proper layering of the solution. If prior CAT scan indicates extensive disease, the procedure could be done under CAT scan to ensure proper needle placement (figures 8-3A and 8-3B).

Predictability of success with prior local-anesthetic blocking

Before neurolytic blocks are performed, a diagnostic local-anesthetic block is usually done a day or so prior to neurolysis. This affords the patient the luxury of feeling the numbness associated with a block and of accepting or rejecting any accompanying side effects. It also affords the anesthesiologist a chance to evaluate the amount of decreased pain experience and the behavior of the patient with the temporary block. Semiquantitative pain scales (such as the Visual Analog Scale for Pain) [27] and sensory/motor testing should be done periodically before and after the local anesthetic block. Incomplete pain relief with local-anesthetic blocking may make the patient reject subsequent neurolysis. Unfortunately, pain relief with local anesthetic is more profound than that with neurolytic agents blocking the same dermatome

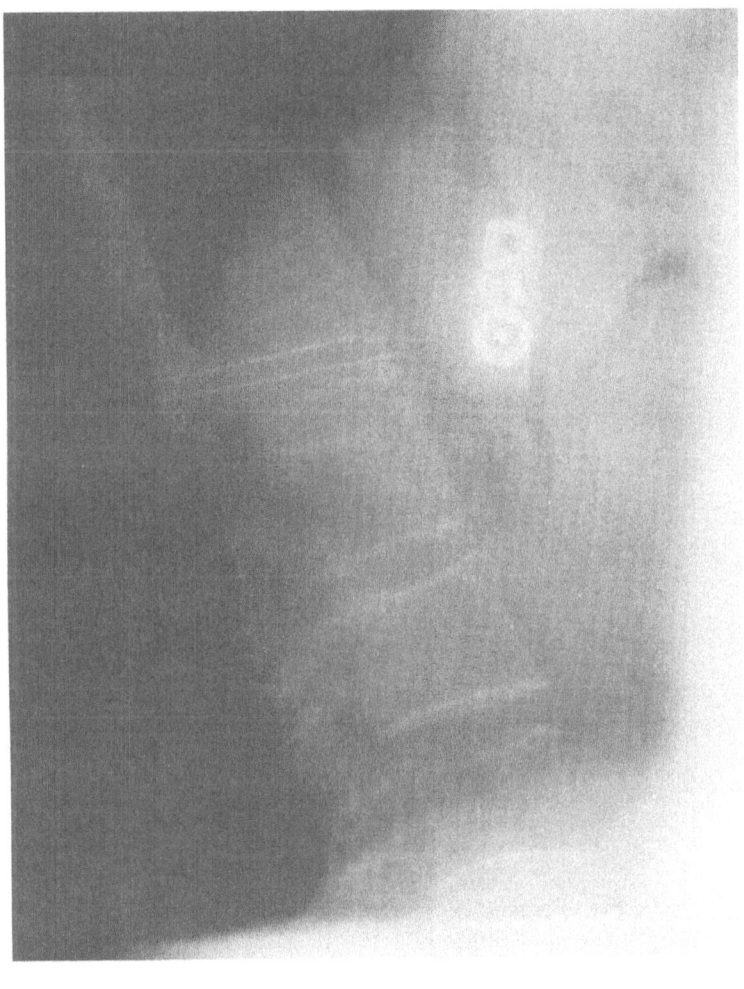

A

Figure 8-2A and 8-2B. Lateral view of needle placement for celiac plexus block before (2A) and after (2B) injection of 5cc of air showing layering in the anterior part of vertebral bodies.

distribution [28]. This is probably due to the possibility that local anesthetics are more diffusible than phenol in penetrating neural tissue. Therefore, a patient who has complete pain relief with a diagnostic local-anesthetic nerve block may not have as profound pain relief after neurolytics.

Changes in pain experience

After a successful neurolytic block, one expects a rapid decrease of pain experience in the cancer patient. However, studies have failed to examine whether these decreased-pain reports are secondary to diminished sensory experience of pain alone or

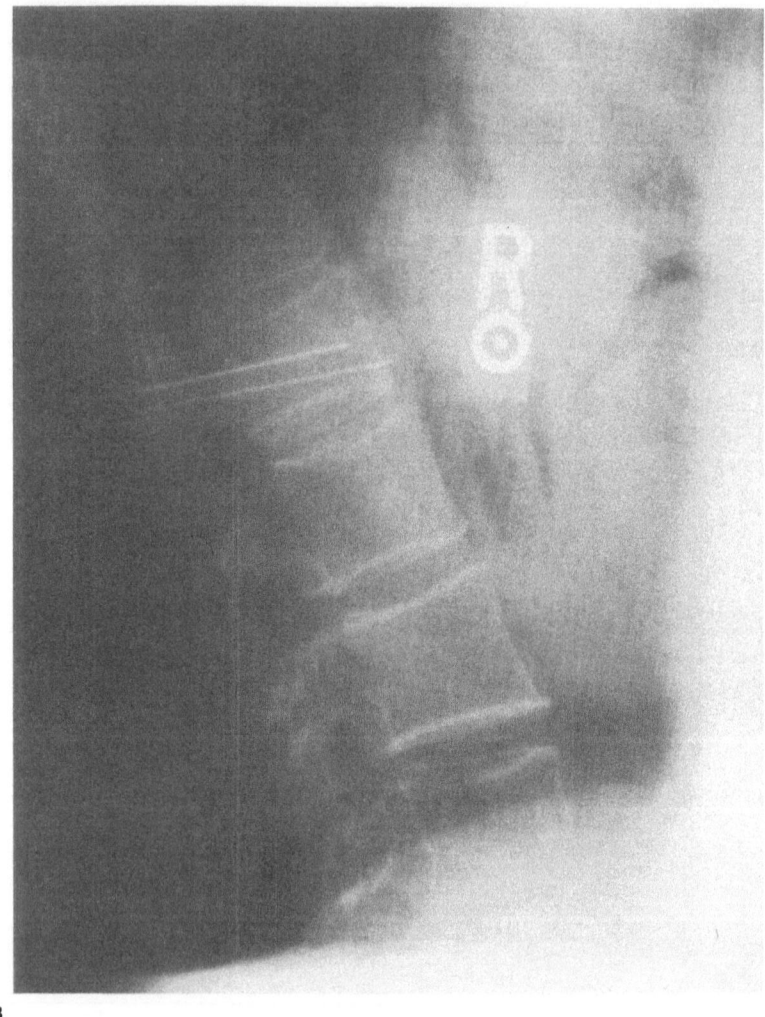

B

whether decreased-pain reports are associated with decreases in the sensory and emotional dimensions of pain experience. The McGill Pain Questionnaire is a paper and pencil type test that can look at both of these dimensions [29].

In our recent pilot study in 92 patients who received neurolytic blocks, only the sensory dimension of pain was significantly decreased in patients who had more than 50% pain relief (figure 8-4), while the affective dimension of pain experience was not decreased at all [30] (figure 8-5). This simply shows that cancer patients receiving neurolytic blocks may have decreased pain experience primarily by decreasing the sensory dimension of pain experience. However, since the affective dimension is not

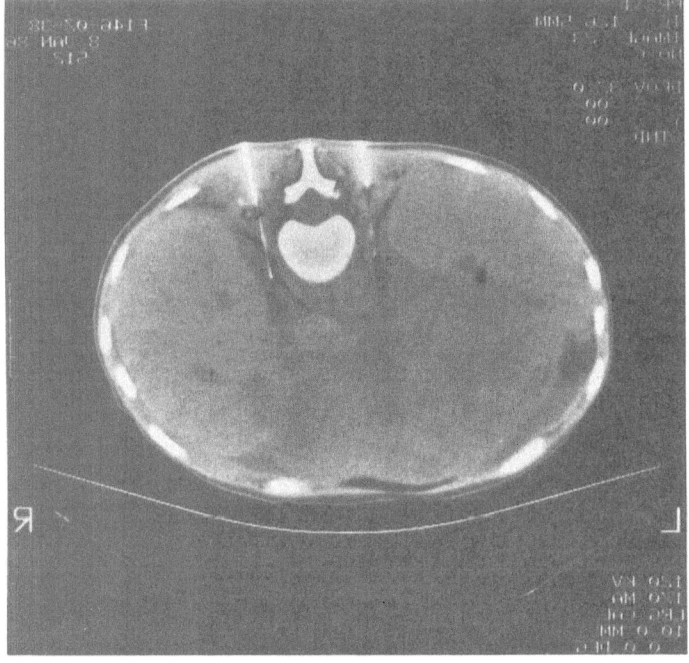

A

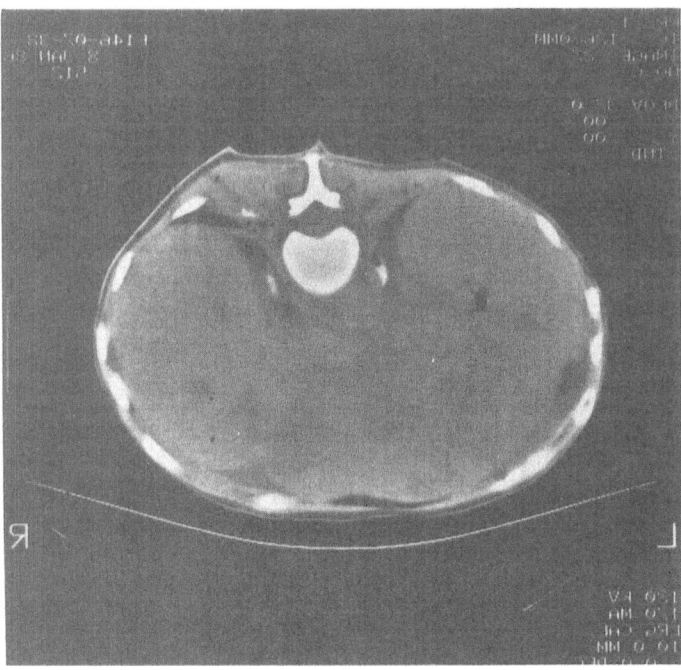

B

Figure 8-3A and 8-3B. CAT scan view of needle placement before (3A) and after (3B) contrast medium injection for celiac plexus block in a patient with extensive disease occupying the entire abdominal cavity.

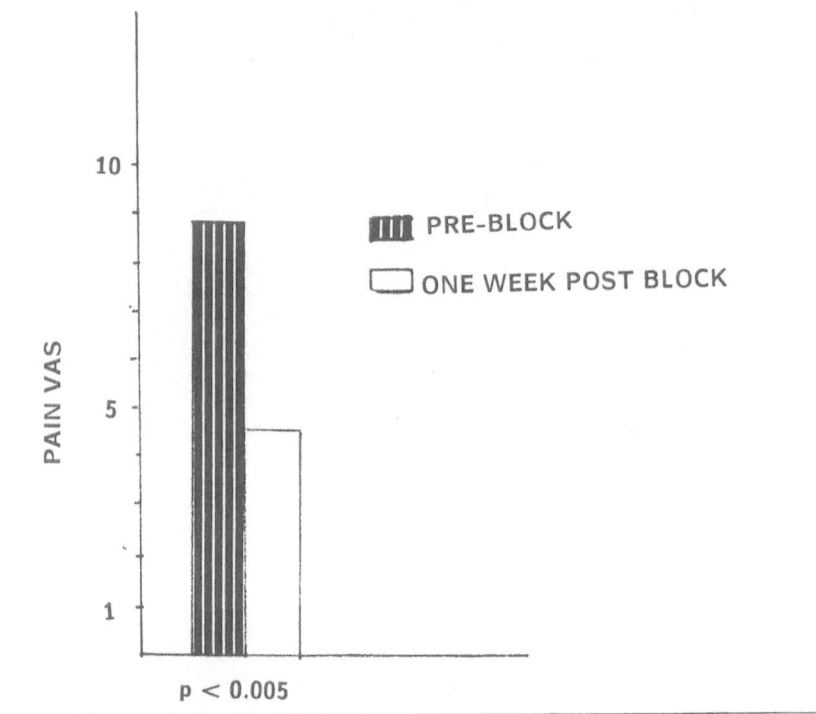

Figure 8-4. Pas VAS in 92 patients with cancer pain, before and one week after neurolytic block, indicating significant, but not complete pain relief.

decreased, the patient may eventually express pain in terms of suffering and hopelessness. This finding emphasizes the continuing importance of incorporating psychological evaluation and management of cancer pain with presently available physical modalities for effective cancer pain management.

Permanence of neurolytic blocks

Most physicians referring cancer pain patients to pain clinics have a myth that neurolytic blocks are permanent solutions to the patient's pain. Neurolytic agents are by no means permanent, since their duration has been reported to be primarily weeks to months at the most [4]. Clinical observations in our institutions confirm these findings. In 15 patients who received thoracic epidural injection in our institution, close monitoring of dermatomal block by mapping areas of decreased sensation postblock indicated regression of sensory loss within hours to days of injection of the neurolytic agents [32]. However, this did not correlate with total return of preblock pain, probably signifying continuous block of small nociceptive C-fibers, but not of the large somatic fibers. Further investigations into this area need to be done.

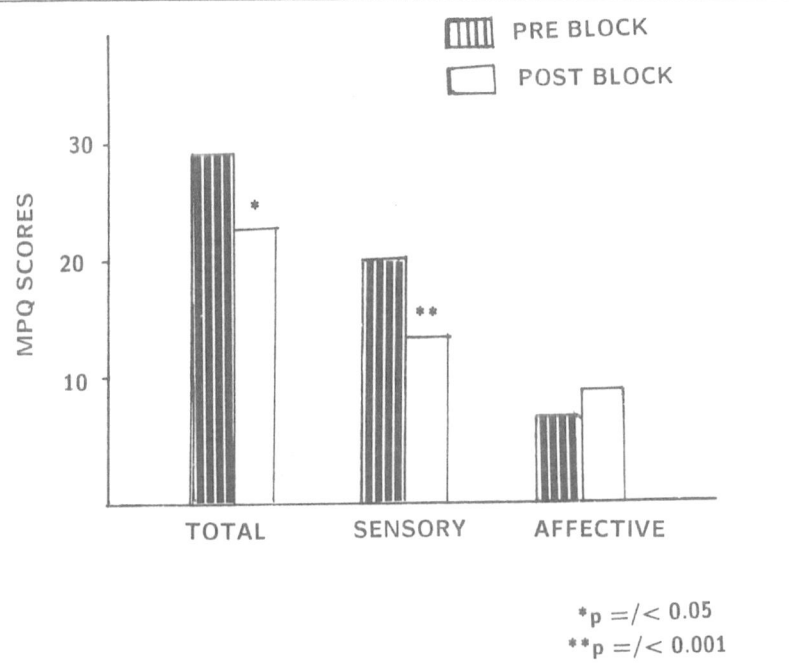

Figure 8-5. MPQ scores in the same 92 patients with cancer pain, before and one week after neurolytic block, indicating significant decrease in sensory dimension, but not in the affective dimension.

POLE OF NEUROLYTIC BLOCKS IN THE MULTIDISCIPLINARY MANAGEMENT OF CANCER PAIN

To maximize optimal pain relief to the patient suffering cancer pain, we need to fully understand the appropriate application of existing modalities for pain management, including neurolytic block. However, inadequate training of physicians, the paucity of easily available information regarding pain control modalities, and lack of specialized resources have hampered adequate application of such modalities. Very few guidelines, other than the appropriate use of narcotic analgesics, have been offered to clinicians involved in the handling of this difficult situation. Recently, efforts have been made to construct a model that rationally integrates various available modalities, including analgesic and adjunctive drug therapy, reduction of tumor size, behavioral–cognitive approaches, mechanical therapy, and neuroinvasive procedures [31]. This model points out several issues that need to be considered before a neurolytic block is considered. First, appropriate drug therapy, with behavioral and mechanical therapy, should be considered before a neuroablative procedure, including neurolytic blocks, is applied. Second, neuroablative procedures should be considered only if there is no pain relief from the above therapies without intolerable side effects (figure 8-6).

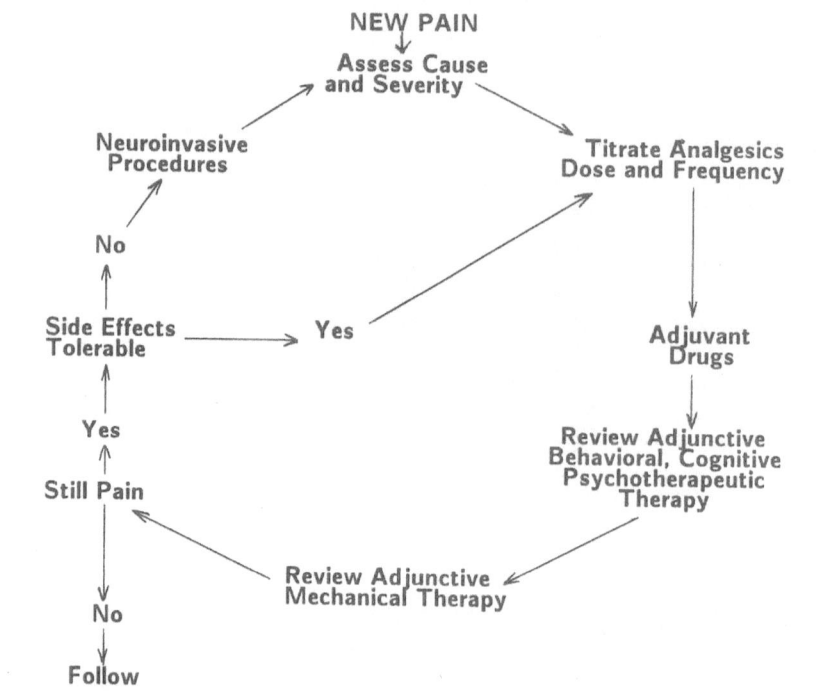

Figure 8-6. Suggested decision tree for the management of cancer pain, incorporating timing for neuroablative procedure (adapted with permission from Cleeland et al. (1986): Journal of Pain and Symptom Management 1:4).

The type of neuroablative procedure is then determined by the extent of the pain (figure 8-7). If localized, the neuroablative procedure is determined by the location of pain. If generalized, the pain is best dealt with by procedures such as deep-brain stimulation [32], hypophysectomy [33], or bilateral chordotomy.

CONCLUSIONS

Neurolytic blocks can be a potent tool for the anesthesiologist to utilize in relieving cancer pain. To maximize their efficacy, we need to understand their appropriate role in the overall multidisciplinary management of cancer pain, given the presently available physical modalities, including pharmacologic, behavioral, and neurosurg-ïcal techniques. The timing of neurolytic blocks is crucial for the cancer patient with pain that may now last from months to years, because of improved life expectancy with current oncologic treatments. We need to look critically at patient selection, indications, and limitations of chemical neurolysis before we proceed with invasive neurolytic block in each individual patient.

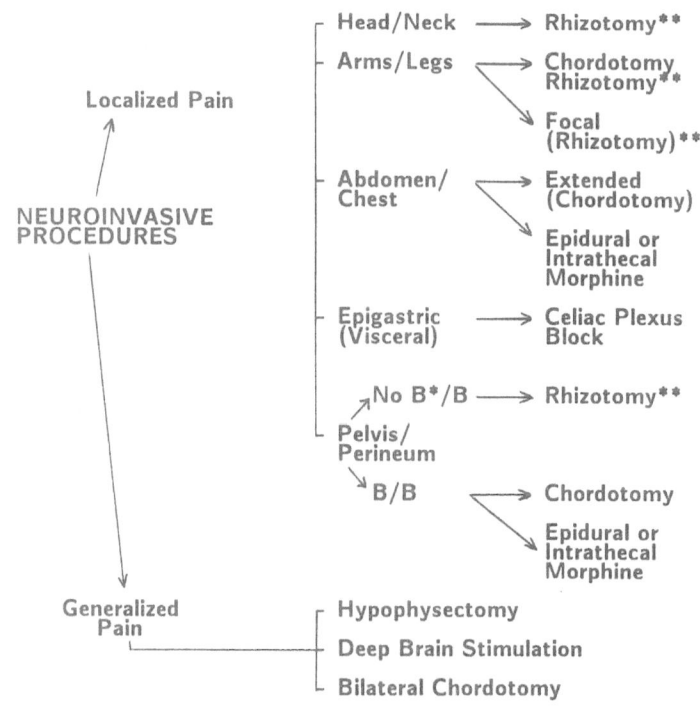

Figure 8-7. Suggested decision tree for neuroinvasive procedures. *Bowel and bladder function; **chemical or surgical rhizotomy (adapted with permission from Cleeland et al. (1986): Journal of Pain and Symptom Management 1:4).

REFERENCES

1. Swedlow M (1974): Relief of Intactable Pain. Amsterdam: Excerpta Medica.
2. Wang JK, Nauss LE, Thomas JE (1979): Pain relief by intrathecally applied morphine in man. Anesthesiology 50:149–151.
3. Daut RL, Cleeland CS (1982): The prevalence and severity of pain in cancer. Cancer 50:1913–1918.
4. Evans RJ, Mackay IM (1972): Subarachnoid phenol blocks for relief of pain in advanced malignancy. Can J Surg 15:50–53.
5. Ferrer-Brechner T (1984): Treating cancer pain as a disease. In: Benedetti C, Chapman C, Morricca G (eds), Advances in Pain Research and Therapy. New York: Raven Press, pp 575–591.
6. Ferrer-Brechner T (1985): The management of pain associated with malignancy. Seminars in Anesthesia 4(4):313–322.
7. Brechner T (1981): Percutaneous cryogenic neurolysis of the articular nerve of Lushka. Reg Anaesth (Suppl 1) 6:18.
8. Lund PC (1971): Principles and Practice of Spinal Anesthesia. Springfield, IL: Charles C. Thomas.
9. Swedlow M (ed) (1974): Relief of Intactable Pain. Amsterdam: Excerpta Medica.
10. Hand LV (1944): Subarachnoid ammonium sulfate therapy for intractable pain. Anesthesiol. 5:544.
11. Ferrer-Brechner T (1981): Epidural and intrathecal phenol neurolysis for cancer pain. Anesthesiol Rev 8:14–19.
12. Cousins MJ, Reeves TS, Glyrin CJ, Walsh JA, Cherry DA (1979): Neurolytic lumbar sympathetic blockade duration of denervation and relief of rest pain. Anesthes Intensive Care 7:121–135.

13. Nathan PW, Scott TG (1958): Intrathecal phenol for intractable pain: Safety and danger of the method. Lancet 1:76.
14. Thompson GE, Moore DC, Bridenbaugh LD, et al. (1977): Abdominal pain and alcohol celiac plexus nerve block. Anesth Analg 56:1–5.
15. Kuzucu GY, Derrick WS, Wibrur SA (1966): Control of intractable pain with subarachnoid alcohol block. JAMA 195:541.
16. Hitchcock E (1969): Osmolytic neurolysis for intractable faceal pain. Lancet 1:434.
17. McKean MC, Hitchcock F (1968): Electro-cardiographic changes after intrathecal hypertonic saline solution. Lancet 2:1083.
18. Ventafridda V, Spreafico R (1974): Subarachnoid saline perfusion. Adv Neurol 4:447.
19. Lucas JT, Ducker TB, Perok PL (1975): Adverse reaction to intrathecal saline injection for control of pain. J Neurosurg 42:557.
20. Ford DJ, Phero JC, Dinson D (1980): Effect of pitcher plant distillate on frog sciatic nerve. Reg Anaesth 5:16–18.
21. Hand LV (1944): Subarachnoid ammonium sulfate for intractable pain, Anesthesiology 5:354.
22. May O (1912): Functional and intragangliones injections of alcohol. Br Med J 2:365.
23. Labat G (1933): Effect of alcohol on the living nerve. Curr Res Anesth Analg 12:190.
24. Ferrer-Brechner T (1986): Anesthetic management of cancer pain. Semin Oncol 12:431–437.
25. Ferrer-Brechner T (1985): The management of pain associated with malignancy. Semin Anesthes 4(4):313–322.
26. Brechner T, Brechner V (1976): Accuracy of needle placement during diagnostic and therapeutic nerve block. In: Bonica JJ, Albe-Fessard D (eds), Advances in Pain Research and Therapy vol 1. New York: Raven Press, pp 679–683.
27. Revill SI, Robinson SO, Rosen M, et al. (1976): The reliability of a linear analog for evaluating pain. Anesthesiology 31:1191.
28. Ferrer-Brechner MT: Unpublished data, 1986.
29. Melzack R (1975): The McGill pain questionnaire: Major properties and scoring methods. Pain 1:277–299.
30. Ferrer-Brechner T, Cohen RS (1984): The role and timing of neural blockade in the multidisciplinary management of cancer pain. In: Gomez Q, Egay L, de la Cruz-Odi M (eds), Anaesthesia—Safety for All. Amsterdam: Elsevier, pp 381–386.
31. Cleeland C, Rotundi A, Brechner T, et al. (1986); A model for the treatment of cancer pain. Journal of Pain and Symptom Management 1:209–215.
32. Young R, Ferrer-Brechner T (1986): Electrical stimulation of the brain for relief of intractable pain due to cancer. Cancer 57:1266–1272.
33. Levin AB, Katz J, Benson RC (1980): Treatment of pain of diffuse metastatic cancer by sterotoxic chemical hypophysectomy: Long-term results and observation on mechanism of action. Neurosurg 6:258–262.

9. ABLATIVE NEUROSURGICAL PROCEDURES IN PAIN RELATED TO MALIGNANCY

PATRICK R. WALSH M.D. PH.D.

Neurosurgical procedures may ameliorate otherwise intractable cancer pain, improve the quality of life, and reduce, or even eliminate, the need for narcosis. A wide variety of ablative and augumentative neurosurgical options exists; each procedure is defined by specific indications, strengths, and limitations. Patient selection is of paramount importance, for in no other clinical situation is the multidimensional nature of pain more apparent than in the setting of malignancy [1,2]. Preexisting fear of unrelenting pain from malignancy may be intense [3], and suffering may be compounded by the depression and anxiety [4] that attend verification of mortality; disability may be more clearly related to angst, to treatment, and to pain than to tumor burden [5,6]. If suffering is primarily a function of anxiety and depression, surgical procedures directed toward interruption of neural pain pathways are destined to fail to afford relief. Similarly, pain arising from nonmalignant sources is rarely appropriately addressed by ablative procedures in patients with cancer.

In addition to definition of the relative contributions of pain, anxiety, and depression to the suffering of the individual with malignancy, effective pain treatment requires a degree of sophistication in identification of the pathophysiologic mechanisms responsible for generation of specific acute, chronic, and mixed pain syndromes at a variety of anatomic locations [7,8]. Psychosocial considerations notwithstanding, multiple specific pain syndromes have been delineated; Turnbull [9] has defined nine different pain syndromes associated with carcinoma of the cervix, in which the results of cordotomy vary dramatically. Although basic pathophysiologic mechanisms remain speculative and controversial in many areas of clinical practice, the attempt should be made to catalogue pain syndromes with appropriate etiologic and descriptive qualifiers that communicate much more effectively than the generic term *cancer pain* and may aid in generation of rational protocols for treatment.

The goal of treatment of pain associated with malignancy is maximal reduction of engendered suffering with the smallest possible risk to the patient and with minimization of treatment-related side effects. Nonnarcotic analgesics and tricyclic antidepressants may contribute substantially to pharmacologic management [8], and narcotic usage reflective of current understanding of pharmacokinetics [10] in a program of escalating narcotic efficacy, as proposed by the World Health Organization [11,12], improves the likelihood of generation of adequate pain relief. Steroidal or chemical neurolytic injections in the hands of an interested and experienced pain-clinic staff may reduce or eliminate the need for continued pharmacologic management. Hospital admission may generate sufficiently detailed medical and neurologic evaluation to delineate relative contributions of various factors to suffering. Attendant manipulation of the regimen of analgesic and adjunctive medications coupled with anesthetic procedures and behavioral intervention may obviate the need for surgery in a large percentage of patients referred for neurosurgical ablative procedures. Such has been the case in approximately 60% of the patients referred to the author for these procedures.

The role of ablative neurosurgical procedures in management of cancer pain is clearly only palliative and has not been well defined; such procedures are often considered only after failure of pharmacologic management to alleviate pain in the debilitated or frankly moribund patient. These characteristics of the population referred for surgical control of pain have been impediments to the generation of large, well-controlled and long-term studies of efficacy of surgical procedures. Nonetheless, effective palliation has been reported to regularly attend surgical maneuvers in intractably afflicted individuals with short life expectancy for whom pharmacologic measures have failed. The limitations and risks of surgical procedures have been well identified; the primary shortcoming of ablative procedures has been the duration of symptomatic relief. Although neurosurgical participation in cancer pain management appears to vary substantially between institutions, Foley [8] and others have suggested that these patients are most effectively treated by a multidisciplinary approach; a neurosurgeon interested in the management of cancer pain may contribute substantially to a multidisciplinary team of oncologists and pain-clinic staff members through earlier consideration of both ablative and augmentative surgical options. The personal experience of the neurosurgeon with various procedures and the oportunity for direct examination of the patient may provide the team with a more realistic understanding of the success of surgical options under consideration than would review of the literature in isolation. Neuroaugmentative procedures [13–17] or narcotic delivery systems [18,19] are generally considered prior to ablative procedures, which are permanent and irreversible and in which duration of analgesia may be disappointingly short.

Pain is a symptom rather than a specific disease, and successful management by ablative surgical techniques is predicated on an understanding of afferent systems and of the central neural pathways and mechanisms in which normal function is to be disturbed. Remarkable advances in the neurosciences have occurred; however, substantial questions remain unanswered. The reader is referred to cogent discussions of neural mechanisms of pain by Bowsher [20] and by Willis [21]. Clinical observations have frequently provided impetus to investigations in the laboratory, and a brief review of pertinent neuroscientific findings will attend the discussion of specific ablative procedures that follows.

Surgical procedures that accomplish cure of malignancy or that deal with pain arising from nonmalignant factors reside beyond the boundaries of this limited presentation, which seeks to outline available surgical options and to summarize related indications and limitations rather than to detail minute technical differences between surgical approaches. The reader is directed to reports of authors with greater experience with individual procedures; when feasible, review articles rather than primary sources have been cited in this presentation. *Pain And The Neurosurgeon—A Forty-Year Experience* by White and Sweet [22] is highly recommended to the reader as a chronicle of thoughtful experience in neurosurgical management of pain.

The primary palliative neurosurgical ablative procedures employed in the management of pain related to malignancy may be divided into four major categories: deafferentation, central disconnection, and neuroendocrine and psychosurgical manipulations. In the first of these options, primary afferent neurones are lesioned either in the peripheral nervous system or at or near the point of entrance of central processes to the spinal cord or brain stem. A number of ablative procedures have been developed to interrupt central pathways that play a role in nociceptive processing; these procedures are perhaps more correctly viewed as affording central disconnection than deafferentation in that primary afferent neurons are preserved. The category of neuroendocrine manipulation in the realm of ablative procedures includes hypophysectomy and interruption of the hypophyseal stalk. Although gratifying results have been reported [22–25] with psychosurgical procedures [21–24], they currently are seldom considered for management of pain related to malignancy [26]. Specific procedures are chosen on the basis of type and location of pain and the clinical status and projected life expectancy of the patient. In all cases, a malignant etiology of pain is assumed, as is persistence of pain despite optimal nonsurgical management. Local irradiation and stabilization when appropriate provide initial options in syndromes of pain related to osseous instability, such as that evidenced in vertebral metastasis with collapse. Persistent pain related to curative surgical or oncologic manipulations is perhaps best approached as benign pain.

Deafferentation procedures employed in management of pain related to malignancy entail division of either peripheral nerves (neurotomy) or of nerve roots (rhizotomy). Diagnostic nerve block with local anesthetic may provide reliable information for surgical planning of neurotomy; although initial postoperative relief of pain has been observed, recurrence is typically rapid and deafferentation phenomena [27,28] are not uncommon. Lesions of mixed peripheral nerves or of mixed dorsal and ventral roots engender motor deficit as well as sensory interruption; such procedures for somatic, noncranial pain ma be effective in the relatively uncommon setting of pain occurring in the distribution of solitary, or a limited number of primarily sensory, peripheral nerves. An extremely useful approach to the management of patients with pelvic malignancy and intractable perineal pain entails division of the sacral nerve roots via extradural ligature through sacral laminectomy [29]. Ventral motor rootlets are sacrificed, and preservation of sphincteric function requires preservation of the S2 nerve root at least unilaterally; the procedure may be carried out caudal to S1 in patients with absent sphincteric function.

Primary deafferentation for somatic, noncranial pain is most often accomplished through selective interruption of dorsal nerve roots which correspond fairly well to sensory systems. Selective dorsal rhizotomy offers the advantage over peripheral neurectomy and chemical rhizotomy of preservation of motor function. At least two roots cephalic to and caudal to the levels involved with pain must be sectioned [26]. Diagnostic nerve root blockade with local anesthetics may assist in surgical planning by determination of both the level and number of dorsal roots involved in pain transmission, and intraoperative somatosensory evoked-potential monitoring may afford direct intraoperative validation. The results of rhizotomy vary widely among investigators [29–33], perhaps in reflection of differences in syndromes approached, technique, tolerance of patients to deafferentation, and duration of survival of patients. Section of insufficient roots or progression of disease dictate persistence or recurrence of pain. Extensive dorsal rhizotomy may render a limb essentially useless with sensory ataxia and may generate unpleasant sensations; however, more limited rhizotomy has been associated with pain relief in selected patients [22]. Failure to accomplish analgesia by selective dorsal rhizotomy may be related to presence of afferent fibers in ventral rootlets [34] or to section of an insufficient number of overlapping dorsal roots; late recurrence of pain after initial analgesia may be related to these factors or to neuroplastic phenomena. Extensive dermatomal overlap [22,35] often dictates the need for a surprisingly extensive laminectomy to permit selective dorsal rhizotomy at a sufficent number of levels to afford relief of pain and may eliminate this option for the debilitated patient. Dysesthesiae may develop several months after traumatic [27,28], chemical, or surgical primary deafferentation; these procedures may therefore be of greatest value in patients with relatively short life expectancy.

The utility of sympathectomy in management of pain associated with malignancy is difficult to estimate through the literature; however, such procedures may be in order if repeated diagnostic blockade affords temporary relief. Non-malignant pain related to primary deafferentation has been approached by Nashold [28] with lesions in the dorsal root entry zone. This approach may constitute an appropriate option in selected patients with deafferentation pain associated with treatment of malignancy or with frank cancer pain.

Craniofacial pain at isolated sites due to tumor may be addressed by either chemical or surgical peripheral neurectomy in occasional cases; however, the distribution of such tumors seldom permits such limited intervention, and rhizotomy is more frequently employed. Trigeminal [36,37] or glossopharyngeal [38] rhizotomy or tractotomy may be accomplished by either open or percutaneous techniques. Section of multiple nerve roots is perhaps of greatest use in approaching intractable pain associated with craniofacial malignancy and may be carried out through posterior fossa craniectomy in sufficiently robust patients [22,39,40]; cranial nerves V, intermedius, IX, and upper X and upper cervical roots may be sectioned. The magnitude of this procedure is obvious, and although pain relief has been reported, medullary [41] tractotomy or more central lesions have been suggested for these patients.

The most complex and voluminous group of ablative neurosurgical procedures involves disconnection of central neural pathways by cordotomy, tractotomy, thalamotomy or cortical ablation. The majority of fibers of the anterolateral fasciculus of the spinal cord terminate in the medullary reticular system [42,43]; smaller numbers terminate in interlaminar thalamic nuclei as the paleo spinothalamic system of Mehler or in the ventrobasal thalamic nuclei as the neospinothalmic system [44]. The role of spinal reticular fibers in nociception is not entirely clear; commisurotomy in animals elicits evidence of only minor input to medullary reticular systems despite the efficacy of this procedure in generation of segmental analgesia [45]. The overall results of these and various pharmacologic investigations are compatible with consideration of paired afferent systems in the anterolateral fasciculus as a polysynaptic spinoreticulodiencephalic system with intralaminar thalamic termination coexisting with a more recently evolved neospinothalamic system that terminates in the ventrobasal thalamic nuclei and generates collaterals to the mesencephalic periaqueductal grey. Anatomic separation of these systems occurs at medullary levels since the neospinothalamic system courses laterally whereas the paleospinothalamic system ascends more medially. Laboratory and clinical findings lend support to tentative assignment of nociceptive conduction and perhaps of chronic pain to fibers of the polysynaptic system and suggest at least some role of the neospinothalamic system in nociception and in suppression of pain [20]. Advantage of the anatomic separation of these systems is taken by ablative tractotomies performed at medullary and more cephalic levels. The complexity of the clinical situation is evident in the findings of Moossy [46] of lesions limited to the dorsal columns at autopsy of patients who had undergone percutaneous cordotomy with reported relief of pain.

Thorough discussions of interruption of the anterolateral spinal fascicular system by cordotomy by open [47–49] and by percutaneous [50,51] techniques are highly recommended to the reader. Cordotomy is typically carried out at either upper cervical or thoracic levels and predictably affords contralateral analgesia; however, the initial cephalic limit of the analgesic zone reflects ascent of several segments of entering fibers before decussation and is therefore several spinal segments caudal to the level of cordotomy. The cephalic limit of the analgesic zone descends over a period of days and often the ultimate analgesic zone is surprisingly small. Detailed observations on this phenomenonon are outlined by White and Sweet [22], who nonetheless chronicled prolonged periods of analgesia. Nathan and Smith [52] correlated the duration of analgesia to the extent of the cordotomy lesion and ascribed recurrence to inadequate section; however, the figure for recurrence of pain at one year in most series is in the range of 50%, despite initial relief in 70–90%. Postoperative development of ipsilateral pain in 10% of patients reflects progression of malignancy or perhaps increased prominence of previously apparently insignificant pain, and may be addressed by the techniques outlined above or by contralateral cordotomy. For the patient with a limited life expectancy, complete relief of pain without need for pharmacologic treatment may represent ideal palliation.

The level of cordotomy is selected on the basis of the distribution of pain. Cervical cordotomy may afford analgesia in the contralateral upper extremity [51,52]. However, due to afferent ascent prior to decussation, White and Sweet were not optimistic about maintenance of analgesia of the arm with this procedure and have noted that neither upper nor mid-cervical pain is predictably ameliorated [22]. The open procedure is typically carried out at the thoracic level to deal with pain exclusively limited to the lower extremities; cervical cordotomy may be chosen for pain with extension to more cephalic levels. Bilateral cordotomy is typically staggered by two spinal segments to avoid the approximately 15% incidence of bladder dysfunction that otherwise may occur. Bilateral cordotomies are usually carried out at T2 to avoid respiratory insufficiency or sleep apnea. These procedures are relatively ineffective in dealing with pelvic pain, for which sacral rhizotomy (described above) appears to be a better procedure. The efficacy and duration of effect of percutaneous cordotomy, initially described by Mullan [53], appears to exceed these parameters for open cordotomy [54]; percutaneous cordotomy clearly constitutes a lesser physiologic stress in the severely debilitated patient.

Additional central disconnective procedures have been directed at diverse tracts and nuclei within the brain stem and in specific situations at cortical sites. Medullary tractotomy has been proposed to extend the cephalic limit of analgesia beyond that attainable with cervical cordotomy, which as noted above is ineffective for cervical pain [22,26,55]. Commissurotomy has been proposed to interrupt spinothalamic crossing fibers at spinal levels to afford a suspended, bilateral segment of analgesia and has become technically feasible with microneurosurgical methods. However, it has not seen widespread use. King [56] outlined advantages of the technique over bilateral cordotomy and reported pain relief in nine patients with late recurrence in two. Mesencephalic tractotomy produces a more cephalic level of analgesia than cervical cordotomy and relief of pain in brachiofacial segments has been reported [57]. Theoretically, a more direct approach to the anatomically focused thalamopetal fibers is afforded with this procedure than with tractotomy performed at more caudal levels. This procedure is exclusively carried out stereotactically, and considerations such as electrode trajectory are reported to reduce the incidence of extraocular motility disorders. Although certain investigators have reported poor results with mesencephalic tractotomy, results reported by Nashold [57] led him to consider mesencephalic tractotomy to be the procedure of choice in brachiofacial pain related to malignancy. Mazars et al. [58] similarly reported consistent relief of pain and considered mesencephalic tractotomy to be the procedure of choice for patients with malignant pain in the upper half of the body on the basis of 216 unilateral and eight bilateral procedures; cordotomy was recommended for lower segmental pain.

A variety of thalamic nuclei have been proposed as lesion sites for dealing with pain associated with malignancy [22,59–64]. The ventrobasal somatosensory thalamic nuclei were approached in early stereotactic procedures and constitute a primary site of termination of fibers of the neospinothalamic component of the anterolateral spinal fascicular system [44]; however, development of *central pain* and sensory loss with ataxia and inconsistent analgesia led to extension of lesions to interlaminar targets [62]. Interlaminar nuclei, including n. centrum medianum and n. parafascicularis, are perhaps the most common targets currently and have somewhat unpredictably generated relief of pain without sensory loss. Central pain has been reported with lesions of the neospinothalamic ventrobasal thalamic nuclei but not with isolated interlaminar lesions. The relationship of specific thalamic nuclear targets to stereotactic landmarks, i.e., the anterior and posterior commissures, is variable, and therefore one must accept cautiously conclusions based on series in which anatomic verification of lesion site is not obtained at autopsy. The extent of lesion beyond specific nuclear boundaries may be substantial, and autopsy verification of the site of lesion has been only inconsistently available. Duration and extent of pain relief have been related to a variety of factors including lesion size and type. Dorsal, medial, pulvinar [64] and anterior [22] nuclear groups have been employed as targets for ablation with variable effects, perhaps in part reflective of cortical connectivity of these nuclei.

Central stereotactic procedures are typically carried out under local anesthesia and therefore may be considered in the relatively debilitated patient and may be repeated when tumor extension occurs [22,61]; however, these procedures are generally considered after failure of other modalities in patients with limited life expectancy due to the often observed rapid loss of analgesia. Electrophysiologic verification of electrode position is commonly employed [65], and these procedures may find more universal usage with the marriage of stereotaxy to CT and MRI localization which obviate the need for operative ventriculography. Descending modulating systems of nociception have not been ablated stereotactically. However, they have been approached for neuroaugmentative procedures [13–17]. Hypothalamic (periventricular nuclei) lesions have been reported to alleviate malignant pain in approximately 70% of patients [66]. It would appear that the majority of current efforts at diencephalic ablative stereotactic relief of malignant pain are directed toward elements of the paleospinothalamic system. However, such lesions frequently extend into neospinothalamic regions.

Cortical resection is rarely carried out for pain associated with malignancy. Central pathways, which are not recognized as primarily nociceptive, have been lesioned in the approach to pain associated with malignancy; these procedures have been for the most part directed toward division of the cingulate bundle [23] or basal frontal cortex [22,24] and are properly considered neuropsychiatric techniques. Neither cingulotomy nor frontal leucotomy appear to be widely employed currently for relief of pain. However, both procedures have been reported to be efficacious in alteration of the perception of pain.

The final category of neural ablative procedures germane to the discussion of management of pain associated with malignancy entails hypophysectomy or section of the hypophyseal stalk. Hypophysectomy was initially carried out through craniotomy via a subfrontal approach. Relief of pain was reported in a high percentage of patients with metastatic breast carcinoma [67] despite the difficulty associated with accomplishing complete hypophysectomy by this approach. Similar results were experienced with section of the hypophyseal stalk. Hypophysectomy is currently most often accomplished by transsphenoidal resection [68], by stereotactic [69] or freehand [70,71] ablation, or by a superior stereotactic approach. Ablation of the gland has been accomplished by stereotactic approaches using a variety of techniques. When neurolytic agents are used, bathing the nuclei of the third ventricle [72] has been reported, as has development of extraocular nerve palsy. It is difficult to explain simply the efficacy of hypophysectomy in relief of pain associated with malignancy on an endocrine basis [68], since pain relief is typically apparent immediately upon awakening from anesthesia, whereas the half-life of TSH and gonadotrophic hormones is substantially longer. ACTH levels are lowered by hypophysectomy and elevated by adrenalectomy; however, both situations may be associated with pain relief, and similar differences are apparent in prolactin levels with pituitary ablation versus stalk section. The lack of predictable effect of naloxone on analgesia suggests no clear role for endorphinergic systems, and analgesia has been reported with incomplete hypophysectomy. Reduction of tumor burden has been reported in approximately one third of patients undergoing hypophysectomy for disseminated malignancy of the prostate or breast and would therefore not provide sufficient explanation for the 90% rate of analgesia reported. Although these procedures have found primary use in endocrine-dependent tumors of the breast and prostate, analgesia has been reported in patients with a wide variety of other tumor types [70].

It should be apparent from this discussion that a number of options exist in the management of pain associated with malignancy; excellent reviews of neurosurgical options are available to the reader [22,73,74]. The sophistication of treatment is a function of the practitioner's appreciation of these options and of the etiology of pain and basis of suffering. Success of symptomatic palliation additionally requires appreciation of normal neural mechanisms to be interrupted for the relief of pain. Perhaps addition of a neurosurgeon or neurologist interested in management of pain associated with malignancy to a multidisciplinary oncologic, behavioral, and anesthetic team would benefit the patient and facilitate earlier identification of options in treatment protocols of patients with various pain syndromes.

REFERENCES

1. Bond MR (1976): Pain and personality in cancer patients. In: Bonica JJ, Albe-Fessard D (eds), Advances in Pain Research and Therapy, vol 1. New York: Raven Press, pp 311–316.
2. Chapman CR (1979): Psychologic and behavioral aspects of cancer pain. In: Bonica JJ, Ventafridda V (eds), Advances in Pain Research and Therapy, vol 2. New York: Raven Press, pp 45–56.

3. Levin DN, Cleeland CS, Dar R (1985): Public attitudes toward cancer pain. Cancer 56:2337–2339.
4. Black RG, Chapman CR (1976): SAD index for clinical assessment of pain. In: Bonica JJ, Albe-Fessard D (eds), Advances in Pain Research and Therapy, vol 9. New York: Raven Press, pp 301–305.
5. Cleeland CS (1984): The impact of pain on the patient with cancer. Cancer 54:263–264.
6. Daut RL, Cleeland CS (1982): The prevalence and severity of pain in cancer. Cancer 50:1913–1918.
7. Foley KM (1979): Pain syndromes in patients with cancer. In: Bonica JJ, Ventafridda V (eds), Advances in Pain Research and Therapy, vol 2. New York: Raven Press, pp 59–75.
8. Foley KM (1985): The treatment of cancer pain. N Engl J Med 313:84–95.
9. Turnbull FA (1959): A basis for decision about cordotomy in cases of pelvic carcinoma. J Neurosurg 16:595–599.
10. Foley KM (1982): The practical use of narcotic analgesics. Symposium on clinical pharmacology of symptom control. Med Clinics of N Amer 66(5):1091–1104.
11. World Health Organization (1986): Cancer pain relief. General Office of Publications, World Health Organization.
12. Ventafridda V, Tamburini M, Caraceni A, DeConno F, Naldi F (1987): A validation study of the WHO method for cancer pain relief. Cancer 59:850–856.
13. Fairman D (1979): Thalamic and hypothalamic stimulation. In: Bonica JJ, Ventafridda V (eds), Advances in Pain Research and Therapy, vol 2. New York: Raven Press, pp 493–498.
14. Larson SJ, Sances A Jr, Reigel DH, Meyer GA, Dallmann DE, Swiontek T (1974): Neurophysiological effects of dorsal column stimulation in man and monkey. J Neurosurg 41(2):217–223.
15. Meyerson BA, Boethius J, Carlsson AM (1979): Alleviation of malignant pain by electrical stimulation in the periventricular–periaqueductal region: Pain relief as related to stimulation sites. In: Bonica JJ et al. (eds), Advances in Pain Research and Therapy, vol 3. New York: Raven Press, pp 525–533.
16. Richardson DE (1979): Central gray stimulation for control of cancer pain. In: Bonica JJ, Ventafridda V (eds), Advances in Pain Research and Therapy, vol 2. New York: Raven Press, pp 487–492.
17. Young RF, Chambi I (1987): Pain relief by electrical stimulation of the periaqueductal and periventricular gray matter. J Neurosurg 66:364–371.
18. Dupen SL, Peterson DG, Bogosian AC, Ramsey DH, Larson C, Omoto M (1987): A new permanent exteriorized epidural catheter for narcotic self-administration to control cancer pain. Cancer 59:986–993.
19. Ventafridda V, Figliuzzi M, Tamburini M, Gori E, Parolaro D, Sala M (1979): Clinical observation on analgesia elicited by intrathecal morphine in cancer patients. In: Bonica JJ et al. (eds), Advances in Pain Research and Therapy, New York: Raven Press, pp 559–565.
20. Bowsher D (1983): Pain pathways and mechanisms. In: Swerdlow M (ed), Relief of Intractable Pain, vol 1. Amsterdam, Elsevier Science, pp 1–23.
21. Willis WD (1976): Spinothalamic system: Physiological aspects. In: Bonica JJ, Albe-Fessard D (eds), Advances in Pain Research and Therapy, vol 1. New York: Raven Press, pp 215–223.
22. White JC, Sweet WH (1969): Pain and the neurosurgeon, a forty year experience. Springfield, IL: Charles C. Thomas.
23. Foltz EL, White LE (1966): Rostral cingulotomy and pain "relief". In: Knighton RS, Dumke PR (eds), Pain. Boston: Little Brown.
24. Freeman W, Watts JW (1950): Psychosurgery in the Treatment of Mental Disorders and Intractable Pain. Springfield, IL: Charles C. Thomas.
25. Hunt RW, Ballantine HT (1974): Sterotactic anterior cingulate lesions for pesistent pain: a report on 68 cases. Clin Neurosurg 21:334–351.
26. Pagni CA (1979): General comments on ablative neurosurgical procedures. In: Bonica JJ, Ventafridda V (eds), Advances in Pain Research and Therapy, vol 2. New York: Raven Press, pp 405–423.
27. Wall PD (1979): Changes in damaged nerve and their sensory consequences. In: Bonica JJ et al. (eds), Advances in Pain Research and Therapy, vol 3. New York: Raven Press, pp 39–52.
28. Nashold BS, Urban B, Zorub DS: Phantom pain relief by focal destruction of the substantia gelatinosa of rolando. In: Bonica JJ, Albe-Fessard D (eds), Advances in Pain Research and Therapy, vol 1. New York: Raven Press, pp 959–963.
29. Crue BL, Todd EM, Wright WH, Maline DB (1970): Sacral rhizotomy for pelvic pain. Pain and Suffering 3:20–24.
30. Pagni CA (1982): Neurosurgical treatment: Status of the problem. In: Bonica JJ et al. (eds), Advances in Pain Research and Therapy, vol 4. New York: Raven Press, pp 165–183.
31. Papo I (1979): Spinal posterior rhizotomy and commissural myelotomy in the treatment of cancer

pain In: Bonica JJ, Ventafridda V (eds), Advances in Pain Research and Therapy, vol 2. New York: Raven Press, pp 439–447.

32. Sweet WH, Poletti CE, Umansky F (1982): Neurosurgical techniques to control the pain of superior pulmonary sulcus and other tumors in this region. In: Bonica JJ, et al. (eds), Advances in Pain Research and Therapy, vol 4. New York: Raven Press, pp 211–233.

33. Barrash JM, Leavens ME (1973): Dorsal rhizotomy for the relief of intractable pain of malignant tumor origin. J Neurosurg 38:755–757.

34. Coggsehall RE, Applebaum ML, Frazen M, Stubbs TB, Sykes MT (1975): Unmyelinated axons in human ventral roots, a possible explanation for the failure of dorsal rhizotomy to release pain. Brain 98:157–166.

35. Foerster O (1933): The dermatomes in man. Brain 56:1–39.

36. Crue BL, Todd EM, Carregal EJA (1970): Percutaneous radiofrequency stereotaxic trigeminal tractotomy. Pain and Suffering Chapter 9.

37. Siegfried J, Broggi G (1979): Percutaneous thermocoagulation of the gasserian ganglion in the treatment of pain in advanced cancer. In: Bonica JJ, Ventafridda V (eds), Advances in Pain Research and Therapy, vol 2. New York: Raven Press, pp 463–468.

38. Broggi G, Siegfried J (1979): Percutaneous differential radiofrequency rhizotomy of glossopharyngeal nerve in facial pain due to cancer. In: Bonica JJ, Ventafridda V (eds), Advances in Pain Research and Therapy, vol 2. New York: Raven Press, pp 469–473.

39. Pagni CA, Maspes PE (1972): The relief of intractable pain in malignant disease of the head and neck by sterotactic thalamotomy or sensory root section. In: Payne JP, Burt RAP (eds), Pain. London: Livingston, pp 204–207.

40. Wetzel N (1966): The relief of pain of malignant disease in the head and neck by sensory root section. Knighton R, Dumke P (eds), London: Churchhill Ltd, pp 431–437.

41. Bricolo A (1979): Medullary tractotomy for cephalic pain of malignant disease. In: Bonica JJ, Ventafridda V (eds), Advances in Pain Research and Therapy, vol 2. New York: Raven Press, pp 453–462.

42. Bowsher D (1957): Termination of the central pain pathway in man: the conscious appreciation of pain. Brain 80:606–622.

43. Mehler WR, Fefferman ME, Nauta WJH (1960): Ascending axon degeneration following anterolateral cordotomy. An experimental study in the monkey. Brain 83:718–750.

44. Mehler WR (1957): The mammalian "pain tract" in phylogeny. Anat Rec 127:332.

45. Kerr FWL, Lippman HH (1974): The primate spinothalamic tract as demonstrated by anterolateral cordotomy and commissural myelotomy. In: Bonica JJ (ed), Advances on Neurology, vol 4. New York: Raven Press, pp 147–156.

46. Moossy J (1969): The pathologist looks at cordotomy. 4th International Congress of Neurology and Surgery. Amsterdam: Excerpta Medica.

47. Brackett CE (1982): Cordotomy by open operative techniques. In: Youmans JR (ed), Neurological Surgery. Philadelphia: W.B. Saunders, pp 3686–3701.

48. Papo I (1979): Open cordotomy in the treatment of cancer pain. In: Bonica JJ, Ventafridda V (eds), Advances in Pain Research and Therapy, vol 2. New York: Raven Press, pp 449–452.

49. Sindou M, Lapras C (1982): Neurosurgical treatment of pain in the pancoast-Tobias syndrome: Selective posterior rhizotomy and open anterolateral C2-cordotomy. In: Bonica JJ et al. (eds), Advances in Pain Research and Therapy, New York: Raven Press, pp 199–206.

50. Lipton S (1979): Percutaneous cervical cordotomy. In: Bonica JJ, Ventafridda V (eds), Advances in Pain Research and Therapy, vol 2. New York: Raven Press, pp 425–437.

51. Rosomoff HL (1982): Stereotactic cordotomy, In: Youmans JR (ed), Advances in Pain Research and Therapy, vol 3. Neurological Surgery. Philadelphia: W.B. Saunders, pp 3672–3685.

52. Nathan PW, Smith MC (1979): Clinico-anatomical correlation in anterolateral cordotomy. In: Bonica JJ et al. (eds), Advances in Pain Research and Therapy, New York: Raven Press, pp 921–926.

53. Mullan S, Harper PV, Hekmatpanah J, Torres H, Dobbin G (1963): Percutaneous interuption of spinal pair tracts by means of a strontium needle. J Neurosurg 20:931.

54. White JC, Sweet WH (1979): Anterolateral cordotomy: Open versus closed comparison of end results. In: Bonica JJ et al. (eds), Advances in Pain Research and Therapy, New York: Raven Press, pp 911–919.

55. Birkenfeld R, Fisher RG (1963): Successful treatment of causalgia of upper extremity with medullary spinothalamic tractotomy. J Neurosurg 20:303–311.

56. King RB (1977): Anterior commissurotomy for intractable pain. J Neurosurg 47:7–11.

57. Nashold BS (1972): Extensive cephalic and oral pain relieved by midbrain tractotomy. Neurol 34:382.
58. Mazars G, Meriene L, Cioloca C (1976): Etat actual de la chirurgie de la doleur. Neurochirurgie (Suppl) 1:1–164.
59. Rodriguez-Burgos F, Arjona V, Rubio E: Stereotactic cryothalamotomy for pain. In: Sweet WH, Obrador S, Martin-Rodriquez JG (eds), Neurosurg Treatment in Psych, Pain and Epilepsy, Baltimore: University Park Press, pp 679–683.
60. Todd EM, Crue BL, Sweet WH, Maline DB (1970): Stereotaxic surgery for relief of pain and suffering. Pain and Suffering 10:81–94.
61. Bouchard G, Mayanagi Y, Martins LF (1977): Advantages and limits of intracerebral stereotactic operations for pain. In: Sweet WH, Obrador S, Martin-Rodriguez J (eds), Neurosurg Treatment in Psych, Pain and Epilepsy. Baltimore: University Park Press, pp 693–697.
62. Mundinger F, Becker P (1977): Long-term results of central stereotactic interventions for pain. In: Sweet WH, Obrador S, Martin-Rodriguez JG (eds), Neurosurg Treatment in Psych, Pain and Epilepsy. Baltimore: University Park Press, pp 685–692.
63. Sano K (1979): Stereotaxic thalamolaminotomy and posteromedia hypothalamotomy for the relief of intractable pain. In: Bonica JJ, Ventafridda V (eds), Advances in Pain Research and Therapy, vol 2. New York: Raven Press, pp 475–485.
64. Laitinen LV (1977): Anterior pulvinotomy in the treatment of intractable pain. In: Sweet WH, Obrador S, Martin-Rodriquez JG (eds), Neurosurg Treatment in Psych, Pain and Epilepsy. Baltimore: University Park Press, pp 669–672.
65. Larson SJ, Sances A Jr (1968): Averaged evoked potentials in stereotaxic surgery. J Neurosurg 28:227–232.
66. Fairman D (1976): Neurophysiological basis for the hypothalamic lesion and stimulation by chronic implanted electrodes for the relief of intractable pain in cancer. In: Bonica JJ, Albe-Fessard D (eds), Advances in Pain Research and Therapy, vol 1. New York: Raven Press, pp 843–847.
67. Ray BS (1967): Hypophysectomy as palliative treatment. JAMA 200:974–975.
68. Tindall GT, Nettleton SP, Nixon DW (1979): Transphenoidal hypophysectomy for disseminated carcinoma of the prostate gland. J Neurosurg 50:275–282.
69. Wright WH, Todd EM, Crue BL, Maline DB (1970): Technique of transnasal stereotaxic radiofrequency hypophysectomy. Pain and Suffering 2:10–19.
70. Moricca G (1976): Neuroadenolysis for diffuse unbearable cancer pain. In: Bonica JJ, Albe-Fessard D (eds), Advances in Pain Research and Therapy, New York: Raven Press, pp 863–866.
71. Lipton S, Miles JB, Williams NE (1979): Pituitary injection of alcohol for inoperable and intractable cancer pain. In: Bonica JJ et al. (eds), Advances in Pain Research and Therapy, vol 3. New York: Raven Press, pp 905–909.
72. Miles J, Lipton S (1976): Mode of action by which pituitary alcohol injection relieves pain. In: Bonica JJ, Albe-Fessard D (eds), Advances in Pain Research and Therapy, vol 1. New York: Raven Press, pp 867–869.
73. Watkins ES (1983): The place of neurosurgery in the relief of intractable pain. In: Swerdlow M (ed), Relief of Intractable Pain, vol 1. Amsterdam: Elsevier Science, pp 305–345.
74. Lee JE (ed) (1977): Pain management. Symposium on the Neurosurgical Treatment of Pain. Baltimore: Williams and Wilkins.

10. MEDICOLEGAL HAZARDS OF DESTRUCTIVE NERVE BLOCKS

CHARLES W. QUIMBY, JR., M.D., LL.B.

The purpose of this chapter is to remind the clinician that, although destructive nerve blocks may bring the patient welcome pain relief, they are dangerous. Their danger stems not only from their anticipated side effect—unwanted concomitant nerve destruction—but also from their unanticipated, unwanted, and unexpected further spread. Unless the clinician impresses on his patient these side effects and the possibility of spread, the clinician is likely to surprise or to anger his patient. It is the surprised or angry patient who is likely to seek redress by legal means—a lawsuit.

For purposes of this chapter, we will tacitly assume not only that the destructive regional block proffered for the management of the terminal cancer patient's pain can manage that pain, but also that the destructive block is in itself dangerous, may have side effects that some patients will find unacceptable, and has complications that are either destructive, unpleasant, or incapacitating to some degree, even when the block is done without error, negligence, or mishap.

Basically, the law is behavioral analysis. Each lawsuit asks: Did the defendant's behavior conform to a given set of criteria or not? The set of criteria used to measure the defendant's behavior can come from either the law of contracts or the law of torts. A *contract* [1] is a consensual agreement between the parties either for the delivery of and payment for goods or for the supplying of and payment for services. A *tort* [2] is a civil wrong. We will be concerned with *assault and battery* (an intentional tort), *informed consent* (an unintentional tort), and *medical malpractice* (an unintentional tort).

CONTRACTS

In the current legal climate, although possible, a suit against a physician for damages for breach of contract for medical services is not likely. However, a suit in contract for breach of warranty [3], or promise to bring about a specific result, is still a possibility. Such a suit can arise when, in his zeal to control the patient's pain, the physician oversells the destructive block.

The law expects the physician to bring his medical training, experience, skill, and expertise to the care of his patient [4]. The clinician should neither promise the patient that he or she will be free of pain nor promise the patient that he or she will feel like his or her old self, nor promise the patient that he or she will have no side effects or complications. Such promises, if made, are likely to be interpreted by both the patient and the courts as a promise to bring about a specified result.

Let us look at language a surgeon used in advising an operation that both the patient and the court thought was a promise to bring about a specified result. In the basic scheme of a contract for services, the offeror offers a service and the offeree accepts those services. Price, although always stated or implied, is not a question here.

Now, when the offeror, with the intent to induce the patient to accept the proffered services, promises that his services will bring about something the patient wants, and the patient, the offeree, accepts these services on the basic of that inducement, the offeror's promise is called a warranty or guarantee [5]. If the inducement, warranty, or guarantee does not come to pass, the contract is broken. This gives the offeree the right to sue the offeror for damages for breach of the contract.

Under a legal analysis, all the offeree, or patient, has to do is show the promise, show its breach, and show the magnitude of the damages. Note: expert medical testimony is *not* needed!

Although *Guilmet v. Campbell* is a suit against a surgeon, one can insert *destructive regional block* for *gastrectomy* and still savor the flavor of this case. The lesson to be learned is this: The physician cannot afford to be a huckster.

The legal issues are (i) Did Dr. Campbell's consultation with the plaintiff constitute a promise to achieve a specific result? (ii) If it did, then did Dr. Campbell's promise induce the plaintiff to undergo the proffered surgical procedure?

Guilmet v. Campbell

385 Mich. 57, 188 N.W.2d 601, 43 A.L.R.3d 1194 (1971)

T.G. Kavanagh, J.—This appeal presents a very simple question . . .

. . . Was the trial court in error in refusing to grant defendant's motion for a judgment notwithstanding the jury's verdict for the plaintiffs?

. . .

The facts and circumstances giving rise to the suit are as follows:

In the fall of 1963 the plaintiff had suffered near fatal bleeding through a peptic ulcer. At that time he was being treated by Dr. Klewicki and it was Dr. Klewicki who recommended the defendant surgeons. In January of 1964 the plaintiff went to see the surgeon "***curious about an operation, if I should have one or if I shouldn't have one***.'' It was never indicated to the plaintiff that he *must* have the operation.

Defendant Dr. Campbell testified that prior to the operation the plaintiff was in excellent physical condition and the operation was *not* an emergency.

At the first consultation with the defendant, Dr. Campbell, the following conversation took place according to the plaintiff's testimony:

Q. Now what was the nature of the conversation? Did you state your purpose in being there?

A. Yes, I asked Dr. Campbell—I was curious about an operation, if I should have one or if I shouldn't have one, I told him. He knew of my records. I started to tell him about my records. He said, 'I know all about your records.' I said, 'Fine.' He told me, he said, '*Once you have an operation, it takes care of all your troubles,*' and he said, '*You can eat as you want to, you can drink as you want to, you can go as you please.*'

Q. This type of operation we are talking about then is a stomach or an ulcer operation, is that right?

A. Yes, it is.

Q. Did you talk with him at all about his familiarity with this type of operation or the extent of the operation?

A. Yes, I did.

Q. What was the conversation as you recall it?

A. Well, he explained to me how they do this operation, and at that time he told me that him and his associate, Dr. Arena, were specialists, *and there was nothing to it at all. It was a very simple operation according to them.*

Q. Did he talk at all about whether he had performed these before?

A. Yes, he did.

Q. And what was the conversation along those lines?

A. I asked him how often. He said, '*Very often.*'

Q. Any discussion as to complications or problems that may arise, that may result?

A. I asked him about it, how long I'd be out of work. He said, 'Approximately *three to four weeks at the most,*' and I asked him about any complications, anything dangerous. He said, '*No, there is no danger at all in this operation.*'

Q. Was there any discussion as to where it would take place, how long you'd be convalescing in the hospital?

A. He said 'Beaumont Hospital.' I'd probably be in four to five days and *then I'd be off work maybe another two to three weeks.*

Q. You say he was familiar with your background. Was he aware that you were taking various medications, Maalox and things of this nature?

A. Yes, he was.

Q. You had been taking these pills for a number of months, had you not?

A. Yes, I had.

Q. What was the discussion about the future use of medication?

A. Well, he said, '*After this operation, you can throw your pillbox away, your Maalox you can throw away,*' and then he come up with an example.

Q. Give the example.

A. The example was that '*In twenty years if you could figure out what you spent for Maalox pills and doctors calls, you could buy an awful lot. Weigh it against an operation.*'

Q. Was there any conversation with him as to operations he had performed on other individuals he had treated for a while?

A. Yes. He told me, he never mentioned no names. He just told me of a gentleman that he knows treated for an ulcer thirty years and he went in, had this operation, *and he is altogether a different man at this time.*

Q. Now at the time of the conversation were you back to work?

A. Yes, I was.

(Emphasis added.)

Following this conversation the plaintiff Richard Guilmet underwent the operation.

The record contains a stark description of the troubles that thereafter befell him.

The record description of the vagotomy reveals activity around and on the esophagus. On March 4, 1964, the day following the operation, Dr. Wood—a specialist in thoracic surgery on the staff of Beaumont Hospital—examined plaintiff and diagnosed: "Ruptured esophagus due to surgical trauma in doing the vagotomy with bilateral effusion and mediastinal emphysema and mediastinitis." Dr. Wood testified that the symptoms displayed by the patient would cause him concern, that the mortality rate from a ruptured esophagus is 50% to 75%.

After the original operation plaintiff went through three subsequent operations for the insertion of tubes to drain excess fluid from his body; he suffered hepatitis which the defendant Dr. Campbell thought was probably caused by one of the many pints of blood he had been given; due to plaintiff's constant coughing and vomiting when eating, his weight fell from 170 pounds to 88 pounds and he was unrecognizable; he was unable to sleep due to coughing and only a return to the hospital and insertion of a drainage tube enabled him to sleep; and finally, he is scarred badly from the operations; he is unable to hold down two jobs as he once could; he is physically weak and unable to be athletically or socially active, and Dr. Wood testified that it is not unusual for recurrences of one of his infections as long as 20 years later.

The plaintiffs brought suit for their damages in a two-count complaint. One count asserted negligence on the part of the defendants in performing the operation, and the other count charged a breach of contract . . .

. . .

The jury returned a verdict of "no negligence" on the tort count but awarded the plaintiffs $50,000 on the breach of contract count.

Justice Talbot Smith [citation omitted] articulated our concern for the sensitivity of this area of engagement, when he said:

"A doctor and his patient, of course, have the same general liberty to contract with respect to their relationship as other parties entering into consensual relationship with one another, and a breach thereof will give rise to a cause of action. It is proper to note, with respect to the contracts of physicians, that certain qualitative differences should be observed, since the doctor's therapeutic reassurance that his patient will be all right, not to worry, must not be converted into a binding promise by the disappointed or quarrelsome."

This sound counsel, however, should not be read to import a different standard to this relationship than to any other. It merely stresses the importance of circumstances in determining the effect of words in establishing a contract. The qualitative difference between the relationship of a physician and his patient and the relationship between a shopkeeper and his customer is a significant circumstance the fact finder must remember in assaying their respective words of undertaking.

As in all contract cases for personal services, in order to find for the plaintiffs here the jury must have found from the evidence that the doctors made a specific, clear and express promise to cure to effect a specific result which was in the reasonable contemplation of both themselves and the plaintiff which was relied upon by the plaintiff.

The plaintiffs say they did, the defendants say they did not.

We conclude that under the circumstances disclosed by this record the trial court was correct in sending this case to the jury to determine the offer, acceptance, breach and damages, and refusing to grant judgment notwithstanding their verdict.

As did the Court of Appeals, we affirm.

ASSAULT AND BATTERY AND CONSENT

Consent [6] is the legal shorthand term for the Anglo–American concept of the inviolability of the individual. In other words, no person shall touch another person without that other person's consent, either express or implied. An illegal touching in our context is a civil wrong in contradistinction to a criminal act. The terms *assault and battery* are used together to describe the prohibited act. *Assault* [7] is the offer of a battery with the present ability to carry out that battery. *Battery* [8] is the touching itself (to batter a person).

Express consent [9] is exemplified by the signed, dated, and properly witnessed surgical consent to operation. A properly drawn, written consent, signed, dated, and witnessed is tangible evidence that can be presented to the court, in case a dispute arises over assault and battery, consent, or its lack.

Implied consent [10] is exemplified by the patient in the examining room who takes off his shirt when the physician says, "I'd like to examine your chest." Although implied consent is equally valid, it is obviously more difficult to establish at trial by oral testimony. But it can be done; otherwise, a patient's clinical record would be stuffed to overflowing with consent forms.

Should the physician, without the patient's consent, touch the patient, examine the patient, or perform a nerve block on the patient, then the physician has exposed himself or herself to a charge of assault and battery. For the defendant physician, the interesting point is that the plaintiff need only show the unlawful touching to prevail at trial! The plaintiff need *not* show injury. If injury is present, all the plaintiff–patient must do is show its presence. No expert testimony of causation is needed. Injury goes only to the magnitude of the money damages the defendant is liable for to the plaintiff.

The upshot of all this is that before the physician performs the block, he should obtain a properly executed consent to the regional block from the patient. The form of the consent must of necessity follow local law and custom. Although its contents and detail are up to the physician, the courts tend to frown on blanket consents as affording the patient insufficient protection. The five journalistic "w's" and, on occasion, "how," will probably satisfy both the patient and the courts. The consent form is tangible evidence to present to the court to defend the physician against a charge of assault and battery.

INFORMED CONSENT [11]

At the outset, let us make it clear that lack of consent and lack of informed consent give rise to two separate and distinct causes of action. The charge of assault and battery arose from the criminal law and is still there. It is an ancient doctrine.

However, assault and battery has been taken into the civil law as an intentional tort. On the other hand, the doctrine of informed consent falls within the purview of negligence (an unintentional tort) and is relatively new.

The essence of negligence is that the plaintiff must have sustained *injury*, an unintentional injury, at the hands of the defendant. In assessing the defendant's fault, negligence uses the following general analysis: The defendant owed a *duty* to the plaintiff; the defendant *breached* that duty; and, as a *direct result* of that breach the plaintiff sustained *injury*. Once the plaintiff has shown the above four items to the satisfaction of the judge, the burden of going forward with the evidence is shifted to the defendant. In other words, the defendant must now defend, justify, or explain his actions.

Although what is injury is sometimes litigated, it is not usually necessary to do so in cases arising from damage due to destructive regional blocks.

In the context of informed consent, the courts have outlined what they think the *duty* should be. Under the doctrine of informed consent, the plaintiff–patient says in effect, "Had the physician informed me of the procedure's complication that has happened to me, which the physician did not, I would not have consented to the procedure."

In an individual case, the physician must fulfill his duty to the patient by telling him or her the procedure's risk or risks. Early in the development of the doctrine of informed consent, the courts started to play the percentage game about what the physician should tell the patient, but soon found that tack wanting.

The courts seem to have come around to a somewhat general but highly applicable and clinically reasonable analysis. The courts feel that, for the patient to be able to effectively participate in decisions concerning his or her health and well-being, the patient needs the following information:

1. Benefits of the proffered procedure;
2. Risks of the procedure, which are the likelihood of
   a. death;
   b. disability;
   c. disfigurement; and,
   d. difficulty in recuperation;
3. The natural history of the disease or problem without the treatment or procedure; and,
4. Alternative treatments or procedures.

Should the patient reject the proffered treatment or procedure and the physician offer another treatment or procedure, the physician should follow the same format for this second recommended procedure. In other words, the physician need only go into the risks and benefits of *alternative* treatments or procedures when they are proffered as a treatment or procedure.

Hales v. *Pittman* illustrates several points. First, it shows how the patient's situation and his instructions to the physician *can enlarge* the physician's obligation to inform the patient. Second, at the time of this case, Arizona had the legal doctrine that *lack of informed consent* rendered the operation or procedure a battery (an intentional tort) rather than a breach of duty, i.e., a negligence action (an unintentional tort), as in most other jurisdictions. Arizona's anomalous view was brought into the majority view by statute "subsequent to the institution of this suit." (Footnote 3, p. 309.)

Hales v. Pittman
118 Ariz. 305 (1978)

Patient, who had undergone phenol injection surgical procedure to eliminate pain caused by tic douloureux, instituted suit against physician alleging, . . . battery . . . when procedure destroyed ophthalmic division nerve fibers. . . . judgment on jury verdict for physician,. and patient appealed. The Supreme Court, Gordon, J., held that: . . . although evidence of physician's previous results in performing surgery was irrelevant to malpractice negligence theory of case, it was relevant to informed consent issue of battery and should have been allowed; . . .

. . .

. . . Dr. Hal Pittman performed a surgical procedure on Leland Hales in order to relieve Hales of the pain caused by tic douloureux, a disease also known as trigeminal neuralgia. Unfortunately, the procedure destroyed the nerve fibers of the ophthalmic division causing the anesthetization of the cornea of the right eye, coupled with a loss of the blink reflex and tearing mechanism. . . . The trial resulted in a defense verdict, and Hales apealed. . . .

. . . At the time of Hales' treatment, at least three methods of treatment were recognized: subtemporal rhizotomy, injections of hyperbaric alcohol or phenol, and radio frequency coagulation. . . .

The probability of an anesthetic cornea occurring varied among the three procedures. Both the subtemporal rhizotomy and radio frequency coagulation presented a five to seven percent chance of an unwanted destruction of the ophthalmic division. Injection of phenol, on the other hand, carried a 23 percent probability of an anesthetic cornea. Of the three methods, the injection of phenol was chosen. Dr. Pittman inserted a 3 1/2 inch needle upward between the right eye and mouth of Hales, injecting .2 cc of phenol. The second and third divisions were immediately anesthetized, and the first division became anesthetic in a few minutes. An additional .1 cc of phenol was then injected to permanently destroy the nerve tissue. Although Dr. Pittman hoped the first division would regenerate and return sensation to the right eye, this never occurred.

. . .

. . . Hales had told Pittman, "Doctor, I can't have anything done to me that's going to interfere with my ability to make a living and support my wife and children." . . . [T]he patient, not the physician, makes the decision on whether to undergo the operation. In other words, if the physician properly informs the patient of the nature and probable results of the operation, as well as alternative methods of treatment, and the patient consents to the operation, . . . the physician is not liable for any unfavorable results. [Citation and footnoes omitted.] . . . [T]he scope of the disclosure required can be expanded by the patient's instructions to the physician. Although the probability of an adverse result may seem slight to the physician, so long as that physician wishes to limit his liability for such results by placing the decision to operate in the hands of the patient, he cannot withhold information if it is relevant to that patient's ability to make an informed consent. Otherwise, by withholding necessary information the physician would usurp the patient's ability to form his own opinion and would, in essence, be making the decision of accepting the non-disclosed risk for the patient. [Citations omitted.] ... Since Hales' wife was an invalid and his children suffered from defective hearing, he deemed his ability to work to be of the utmost importance. He instructed Dr. Pittman of these facts and should have been informed of the risks which could affect his ability to work.... If ... Dr. Pittman failed to provide Hales with sufficient information to allow an informed decision to be made, the law recognizes an action founded on battery....

· · ·

... [A]nything greater or different than the procedure consented to becomes a battery....

· · ·

Evidence of Other Complications
Appellant was not permitted to introduce evidence of Dr. Pittman's previous experience with phenol injections. Prior to the operation on Hales, Dr. Pittman had utilized the same procedure on four patients. Two of these patients, but not Hales, developed a complication known as anesthesia dolorosa. This is a constant pain which is sometimes worse than the tic douloureux which the operation is designed to eliminate. Appellant offered to prove that the failure of Dr. Pittman to inform Hales of these previous unwanted results ... and that had Hales known of these previous results, he would not have consented to the operation....
   ... [T]he unauthorized touching rather than its results technically forms the basis of a battery action.

· · ·

... Battery, however, was also a theory, thereby rendering the evidence of the anesthesia dolorosa incidents relevant. As noted above, without an informed consent by Hales, the operation constituted a battery....

· · ·

... [T]he patient must understand "substantially the nature of the surgical procedure attempted and *the probable results of the operation.*" (Emphasis supplied.) ... To properly weigh the advantages of elective surgery with its attributable disadvantages, a person needs information not only concerning the statistical probabilities of various adverse results ... but also one is entitled to information concerning the treating physician's experience with the particular procedure.... We hold, therefore, that evidence of prior results is relevant to the informed consent issue of battery. Since appellant was prevented from introducing evidence of appellee's previous experience with phenol injections and evidence that the failure to inform Hales of these results, in addition to the general probability of encountering anesthesia dolorosa, fell below the applicable standard of care, the jury could not properly evaluate the battery count. Given these facts the jury could have found that a reasonable person, properly informed would not have consented to the operation. Therefore, the judgment is reversed for a new trial on the question of battery.

The informed consent encounter

From an analytic and objective point of view, the informed consent encounter is a teaching–learning encounter.
   Viewed in this light, the physician's legal obligation (duty) is to teach the patient sufficient clinical medicine for the patient to participate effectively in his or her selecting one or more treatments from among those proffered. In our context, it is the selection or acceptance of the proffered destructive nerve block.
   Unfortunately, this learning encounter is taking place under the worst possible

circumstances. First, the patient already has on his or her mind the impact of the disease and severe pain on self and family. Second, because of his or her terminal illness that he or she knows of or firmly suspects, the patient can be expected to be in a state of denial, anger, depression, or acceptance. Should the patient be denying the terminal illness or be angry about it or depressed over it, the patient's ability to learn often highly technical material and often unpleasant truths is impaired, if not destroyed.

Because the patient is seeking relief of his or her pain, he or she is neither denying it nor accepting it. Furthermore, the patient can also be expected to be angry about the pain, depressed over it, or, perhaps, in a bargaining mood. None of these mental states is likely to enhance learning; rather, they further distract the patient from learning.

Finally, what is the patient's medication status? Is the patient on sedatives? Is the patient on tranquilizers? Is the patient on antidepressants? Is the patient on narcotics? Is the patient addicted to narcotics or dependent on other medications? Any of these drugs may impair the patient's ability to learn.

After taking into consideration all the above questions, as well as the patient's basic personality, background, training, and ability to learn, the clinician must then determine whether or not he will be able to *teach* the patient the appropriate clinical medicine to allow the patient to participate effectively in selecting his or her mode of therapy, here destructive nerve block.

In summary, we have a patient who is distracted by weighty problems of self and family, whose psychiatric status is likely to be one of denial, anger, or depression, and whose medication regimen may be at toxic and addictive levels. It is under these conditions that the clinician is legally obligated to teach this patient highly technical and often unpleasant material.

What is the clinician to do? Obviously the clinician can run the material by the patient. Do it *pro forma*. However, such activity is not likely to pass muster in court.

The clinician might *withdraw* medications early enough before the interview so that the patient is not mentally fogged. Withdrawal of medication has three drawbacks. First, the patient may be so distracted by pain that he is unable to follow the clinician and learn. Second, this tack might be considered an unconscionable lever to force the patient to select the clinician's proffered nerve block. Third, the patient may be starting to have withdrawal symptoms at the time of the interview. All these are counterproductive.

Another avenue of approach might be for the clinician to *adjust* the patient's medications to levels where the patient is not intellectually fogged by medication and yet is comfortable. This implies the patient's primary physician is overdosing the patient at this time. Hence, this avenue is at best tenuous. Finally, the court can say with complete truth, "The patient was under the influence of drugs and could give neither consent nor be sufficiently informed to give informed consent." Although reasonable from a clinical point of view, it is doubtful that this is a safe legal alternative.

The clinician has the option of conducting the informed consent interview with the patient and an appropriate responsible person, such as spouse, family member, parent of adult child as appropriate, or other appropriate person present. We assume the patient is in the optimum condition to listen, learn, and discuss the risks and benefits with the physician. It would seem prudent under these circumstances for the clinician to impart the information, answer questions, and then schedule another interview at a later date with the same participants—the patient and responsible adult. At the second interview other questions can be answered, if any; the patient's decision can be recorded; and, if accepted, the block can be scheduled. This procedure imparts and clarifies the necessary information, allows the patient, whatever his mental status may be, to go over the information, and gives the patient a resource person in the interim, should that person be needed. It also removes any pressure on the patient for a decision.

It should be noted here that the law does not prescribe what shall be told to the patient specifically but only in general terms and the law does not prescribe how the information shall be imparted. There can be an interview, an interview with handout, an interview with slide presentation, an interview with video presentation, or perhaps in unusual cases only a handout, and decision.

How to manage the informed consent encounter is limited only by the clinician's experience and ingenuity as well as his ability to impart the requisite information in view of the patient's status.

Documentation

The reason for this chapter is that the physician may be the defendant, not the plaintiff. As defendant in a suit alleging lack of informed consent, the physician will have to describe his behavior as precisely as he can, justify that behavior, and convince the court, judge or jury, or both that his behavior meets the legal criteria. This can be done by oral testimony or by written evidence or by both.

Oral testimony relying on memory is a sometime thing. Memory is known to fade, change over time, and be subject to the vantage point of the one testifying. All this is not to deprecate oral testimony relying on memory, but to place it in its proper perspective.

Documentation of the informed consent encounter and its proper authentication [12] at trial obviates memory or the need for it. The clinician would be well advised to follow the journalistic "five w's" plus "how" to document the informed consent interview(s). *Who* was present and *why*? *What* information was imparted? *What* was the mental status and receptivity of the patient? *When* did the interview take place? This is for correlation with medication, if needed later. *Where* was the informed consent interview held? *How* was information imparted? Verbally? By handout? Slide presentation? Movie or video presentation? Some combination of the above? Tapes, slides, and handouts should be available for the court, if need be.

At trial, the physician's documentation in the patient's chart or for his own files will have to be properly authenticated. This means that the document must be shown to connect its contents with the informed consent interview(s) under scrutiny. This can be done, *subject to one's jurisdictional rules*, by signing the document, dating it, listing who was present and for what reason, and then having it witnessed by one or more disinterested witnesses.

Although some patients want a full informed consent discussion with their physician, other patients want only an abbreviated discussion and still others want no discussion at all, only the treatment or procedure. An important element of the clinician's note is his documentation of which group the patient falls into.

If the patient falls into that group who wish only an abbreviated discussion, the clinician should clearly document this fact and either how it was arrived at or how the patient communicated it to the clinician. From a legal analysis, the abbreviated discussion is quite dangerous for the clinician. If an undiscussed complication or side effect occurs, the patient could claim he or she would not have given consent to the procedure, had he or she only known. A prudent course of action would be for the clinician to state the complications and side effects that were discussed and those areas omitted *and why!* Alternatively, all complications can be told to a responsible adult involved with the patient.

If the patient shows the clinician by words or by actions that he or she does not wish to discuss the side effects and complications of the proposed treatment or procedure at all, the clinician should document the patient's behavior and the fact the patient did not want the informed consent discussion. At this point, depending upon the situation at hand, the clinician must decide whether it is appropriate to have an informed consent discussion with a responsible person, spouse or family member, or some other appropriate responsible adult involved with the patient.

Again, in selected cases prudence would suggest that complete and appropriate information be imparted to the responsible adult involved with the patient. Documentation of this interview is likewise prudent.

MEDICAL MALPRACTICE

Malpractice is negligence in the performance of a professional act [13]. In general, a medical malpractice suit requires the testimony of an expert witness(es) to instruct the court about the professional and technical facts of the case.

Negligence or fault analysis has been distilled over the years to the following paradigm:

The defendant owed a *duty* to the plaintiff; the defendant *breached* that duty; and, as a direct result of that breach (*proximate cause*), the patient was *injured*. Or, more concisely: *Duty, breach, proximate cause*, and *injury*. Without injury there is no negligence or malpractice.

Whereas, in an informed consent suit, the duty has been outlined by the courts, in a suit for medical malpractice the duty must be articulated as dictated by the fact situation under scrutiny. For example, the duty relevant to a malpractice suit about an appendectomy differs from that of a suit about the medical management of an arrhythmia. Expert witnesses are needed to articulate to the court the duty the defendant owed to the plaintiff.

In analyzing a given fact situation *for the potential* of medical malpractice, the clinician ought to articulate *clearly and concisely* for himself the duty or duties the physician owed to the patient, and then ask: Was the duty breached? Did the breach of this duty directly cause the patient's injury? (Alternatively, was the breach of duty the proximate cause of the plaintiff's injury?) If the answer is "Yes" to these two questions, there is a potential for a medical malpractice suit. If the answer to one of these questions is "No" on the basis of the articulated duty, then there is no potential for medical malpractice.

The term *potential medical malpractice* is used to indicate that the defendant is guilty of medical malpractice only after a trial court has found the defendant at fault *and* all appeals have been exhausted.

At trial, the plaintiff, a layman, uses the testimony of his expert witness(es) to present to the court the duty or duties owed to him. The defendant can use the testimony of his own expert witness(es) to articulate the duty(ies) owed to the patient; or, he may act as his own expert witness. The choice is a matter of tactics.

An expert witness's articulation of how to perform a block is an example of testimony that establishes a duty owed to the plaintiff by the defendant physician.

The jury, under the judge's instructions, selects from the proffered competing duties which duty is the proper one for the fact situation under scrutiny. Then the jury must determine whether or not the defendant breached that duty under the facts of the case. The next question they must answer is: Was the breach of duty the direct or proximate cause of the patient's injury? If not, medical malpractice does not exist. If yes, the defendant is said to be at fault or guilty of medical malpractice and liable to the plaintiff in money damages.

From a medical point of view, how to perform a treatment or procedure usually falls into the majority's method or into one or several significant or sizeable minority's method(s). The law does not try to select between the majority or minority(ies) method(s).

At times, one or a very few mavericks have a method all their own. These methods are generally frowned upon by the jury, and more so if the jury feels the method is experimental.

Foil v. *Ballinger*, 601 P.2d 144 is quoted here to give the flavor of judicial thinking about the side effects of destructive nerve blocks. This case was a malpractice action that the trial court dismissed, i.e., it did not go to trial, because the Statute of Limitations had run. The Utah Supreme Court addressed procedural issues. Although the patient was not terminally ill with cancer, the alleged malpractice was about a phenol nerve block.

Foil, the plaintiff, had continued severe back pain following a spinal fusion that extended a prior spinal fusion. The patient consulted an anesthesiologist for his continued back pain. Several caudal anesthetics brought transient relief. The anesthesiologist performed a "permanent subarachnoid phenol block." Following the phenol block, the patient suffered rectal and bladder dysfunction. To rectify these problems, the patient underwent several surgical procedures.

The patient sued the anesthesiologist who administered the phenol block for medical malpractice.

Because of a retroactive procedural statute, the patient instituted his malpractice suit just before and just after the Statute of Limitations had run on his cause of action. The trial court sustained the defendant's defense that the Statute had run. The plaintiff appealed to the Utah Supreme Court.

On appeal, the Supreme Court reversed the trial court's decision. In reaching its decision, the court outlines how it feels about *medical treatment by experts and the layman's comprehension of injury and possible negligence.*

For the physician reader, the court's long sentences and wordiness should not mask what the court is saying.

Foil v. Ballinger
601 P.2d 144 (1979)

. . .

. . . In the health care field it is typically the case that there often is a great disparity in the knowledge of those who provide health care services and those who receive the services with respect to expected and unexpected side effects of a given procedure, as well as the nature, degree, and extent of expected aftereffects. While the recipient may be aware of a disability or dysfunction, there may be, to the untutored understanding of the average layman, no apparent connection between the treatment provided by a physician and the injury suffered. Even if there is, it may be passed off as an unavoidable side effect or a side effect that will pass with time. Indeed, common experience teaches that one often suffers pain and other physical difficulties without knowing or suspecting the true cause, and may, as often happens, ascribe a totally erroneous cause to the manifestations. . . . A number of medical difficulties can readily be attributed by a layman to causes that are known or should be known. But when injuries are suffered that have been caused by an unknown act of negligence by an expert, the law ought not to be construed to destroy a right of action before a person even becomes aware of the existence of that right. [at P. 147]

REFERENCES

1. Restatement, Second, Torts § 1. Contract Defined: A contract is a promise or set of promises for the breach of which the law gives a remedy, or the performance of which the law in some way recognizes as a duty.

   American Law Institute Publishers, St. Paul, Minn., 1965.

2. Restatement, Second, Torts § 6. Tortious Conduct: The word *tortious* is used throughout the Restatement of this Subject to denote the fact that conduct whether of act or omission is of such a character as to subject the actor to liability under the principles of the law of Torts.
   Comment: a. The word *tortious* is appropriate to describe not only an act which is intended to cause an invasion of an interest legally protected against intentional invasion, or conduct which is negligent as creating an unreasonable risk of invasion of such an interest, but also conduct which is carried on at the risk that the actor shall be subject to liability for harm caused thereby, although no such harm is intended and the harm cannot be prevented by any precautions or care which it is practicable to require.

   American Law Institute Publishers, St. Paul, Minn., 1965.

3. Warranty . . . A promise that certain facts are truly as they are represented to be and that they will remain so, subject to any specified limitations.

   Black's Law Dictionary, West Publishing Co., St. Paul, Minn., 1979.

4. Restatement, Second, Torts § 299A. Undertaking in a Profession . . .: Unless he represents that he has greater or less skill or knowledge, one who undertakes to render services in the practice of a profession . . . is required to exercise the skill and knowledge normally possessed by members of that profession . . . in good standing in similar communities.

American Law Institute Publishers, St. Paul, Minn., 1965.

5. See footnote 3 above.

6. (a) Restatement, Second, Torts § 10A. Consent: The word *consent* is used . . . to denote willingness in fact that an act or an invasion of an interest shall take place.
   (b) Restatement, Second, Torts § 892. Meaning of Consent:
   (1) Consent is willingness in fact for conduct to occur. It may be manifested by action or inaction and need not be communicated to the actor.
   (2) If words or conduct are reasonably understood by another to be intended as consent, they constitute apparent consent and are as effective as consent in fact.

American Law Institute Publishers, St. Paul, Minn., 1965.

7. Restatement, Second, Torts § 21. Assault: (1) An actor is subject to liability to another for assault if (a) he acts intending to cause a harmful or offensive contact with the person of the other or a third person, or an imminent apprehension of such a contact, and (b) the other is thereby put in such imminent apprehension. . . .

American Law Institute Publishers, St. Paul, Minn., 1965.

8. (a) Restatement, Second, Torts, § 18. Battery: Offensive Contact:
   (1) An actor is subject to liability to another for battery if
   (a) he acts intending to cause a harmful or offensive contact with the person of the other or a third person, or an imminent apprehension of such a contact, and
   (b) an offensive contact with the person of the other directly or indirectly results.
   (2) An act which is not done with the intention stated in Subsection (1,a) does not make the actor liable to the other for a mere offensive contact with the other's person although the act involves an unreasonable risk of inflicting it and, therefore, would be negligent or reckless if the risk threatened bodily harm.
   Comment: . . . Since the essence of the plaintiff's grievance consists in the offense to the dignity involved in the unpermitted and intentional invasion of the inviolability of his person and not in any physical harm done to his body, it is not necessary that the plaintiff's actual body be disturbed. Unpermitted and intentional contacts with anything so connected with the body as to be customarily regarded as part of the other's person and therefore as partaking of its inviolability is actionable as an offensive contact with his person. . . .
   (b) Restatement, Second, Torts, § 13. Battery: Harmful Contact: An actor is subject to liability to another for battery if
   (a) he acts intending to cause a harmful or offensive contact with the person of the other or a third person, or an imminent apprehension of such a contact, and
   (b) a harmful contact with the person of the other directly or indirectly results.

American Law Institute Publishers, St. Paul, Minn., 1965.

9. Express consent. That directly given, either [orally] or in writing . . .

Black's Law Dictionary, West Publishing Co., St. Paul, Minn., 1979.

10. Implied consent. [Consent] manifested by signs, actions, or fact, or by inaction or silence, which raise a presumption that the consent has been given.

Black's Law Dictionary, West Publishing Co., St. Paul, Minn., 1979.

11. Informed consent: A person's agreement to allow something to happen ... that is based on a full disclosure of facts needed to make the decision intelligently; ...

Ze Barth in Swedish Hospital Medical Center, 81 Wash.2d 12, 499 P.2d 1, 8.

12. Authentication. In the law of evidence, the act or mode of giving authority or legal authenticity to a ... record, or other written instrument, ... so as to render it legally admissible in evidence....

Black's Law Dictionary, West Publishing Co., St. Paul, Minn., 1979.

13. Restatement, Second, Torts, § 282. Negligence Defined: ... [N]egligence is conduct which falls below the standard established by law for the protection of others against unreasonable risk of harm. It does not include conduct recklessly disregardful of an interest of others.

American Law Institute Publishers, St. Paul, Minn., 1965.

11. HOSPICE CARE OF THE CANCER PAIN PATIENT

SHELDON L. BURCHMAN, M.D.

To begin this chapter, we should note that a major problem confronting modern medicine is the need to educate some physicians and nurses. These physicians and nurses must learn that there is a time to forget cure and to be concerned with care. To everything there is a season, and there comes a time when hospital heroics, such as dramatic surgical interventions and continuation of life support systems, make no sense. As hospice expert Sister Harriet Copperman says, "There comes a time when we should ask ourselves, 'In fact, what's wrong with dying?'"

HOSPICE

Give me your tired, your poor,
Your huddled masses, yearning to breathe free,
The wretched refuse of your teaming shore.
Send these, the homeless, tempest-tost to me,
I lift my lamp beside the golden door!

These words of hope inscribed on a tablet in the pedestal of the Statue of Liberty in New York Harbor were written by Emma Lazarus over 100 years ago. The concept of reaching out to illume the way for the downtrodden is embodied in present-day hospice philosophy.

The word *hospice* originated with the medieval Latin *Hospitium*, or *guest house*, which provided for the needs of weary pilgrims. The physical shelter had strongly religious foundations, which St. Benedict so aptly stated: "Hospes venit; Christus

153

venit! When a guest arrives, treat him as though he is the messiah, for well he may be."

Travel in the ancient Near East was hopelessly difficult.

Abraham's travels were made easier by the encounter with Melchizedek who offered him bread and wine. Nearly 2000 years ago Fabiola, a disciple of St. Jerome, cared for pilgrims returning from Africa. The offering of food to the traveler became almost a sacrament in the ancient world as an outward sign of God's presence. In the book of Exodus, God commanded Moses to construct a sanctuary, an emblem that God dwells amongst us. The hospice is that sanctuary and God lives in the hearts of all who enter.

The hospice movement stands as a beacon of sanity in a turbulent and uncaring world. Here once again in the cycle of time, human compassion has been reborn. From biblical times to the present, we have seen a reshaping, remolding, and refining of this hospice concept of God's presence and help to both the dying and the traveler. This concept of hospice took its origins in biblical times.

Prior to World War II, birth and death were commonplace in the home. This author was born at home and watched as a child the death of grandparents in our home. He attended numerous Irish wakes in a mixed Irish–Jewish neigborhood in the Bronx, New York and marveled at the sharing of this journey into the unknown. The sitting or *shiva* in Judaism, which is prescribed after death, represents as in other religions the sharing of the burdens of death.

However, with the advent of widespread health insurance, advanced medical technology, and a hospital-building program of gigantic and unrestrained proportions, hospitals became an acceptable place for the dying. The home was the alien place and the families and friends became shapeless and unwelcome blurs at the bedside; we in the profession pronounced "Nothing more can be done." The hospice is truly the answer to "nothing more can be done." Unfortunately, many hospitals, doctors, and nurses are still not aware of the many advantages of hospice care.

This message of care was and is sorely needed. The deathbed statement of Dr. Frederic Stenn [1] bears shameful testimony to our shortcomings in care. Dr. Frederic Stenn, on his deathbed, wrote the following:

Most physicians have lost the pearl that was once an intimate part of medicine, and that is humanism. Machinery, efficiency and precision have driven from the heart warmth, compassion, sympathy and concern for the individual. Medicine is now an icy science; its charm belongs to another age. They dying man can get little comfort from the mechanical doctor.

The hospice movement has rediscovered and refined the pearl. It, too, like the lamp at the golden door brings hope to the weary traveler and lights the way on this cyclical journey of life.

Dublin in the middle nineteenth century, like the world over, had little time to care for the dying and the sick, and it was to this prevailing indifference that Mary Aikenhead thrust her energies in founding the Irish Sisters of Charity [2]. She viewed death as the beginning of a journey and provided hospice care to those unfortunates who traveled this road. In 1905 she established St. Joseph's Hospice in London, England, and it was to St. Joseph's that Cicely Saunders, a young medical student, came in 1958 to open a window to the world on terminal care. It was to her vision and pursuit of knowledge in the care of the terminally ill that the world owes an eternal debt of gratitude. She successfully wed science and compassion to the extraordinary nursing dedication of the nuns of St. Joseph's Hospice. Her deep faith was evident. While reading from Psalm 37 on June 24, 1959, Dame Cicely Saunders was struck by the phrase "Commit thy way unto the Lord; trust also in him; and he shall bring it to pass." Thus the modern-day era of hospice, the concept of care, and the seeds of St. Christopher were firmly planted in her mind. In 1967 her dream was realized and St. Christopher's Hospice opened its heart and its doors as a community for the dying. It was here that the patient took priority over the disease. It was here that the family was included for the first time as part of a caring concept. Death is accepted, cure fades, as care intensity increases.

Hospice is not a cult of death and dying, nor is it a physical place. It is an emotion, a philosophy, and a concept that permits us to control pain, to ensure general comfort (both spiritual and mental) to assure a dignified death for the patient, and to give support to the family before, during, and after death. There is a breeze of good cheer in the symbiosis between the caring team, the patients, and their families. There is a giving and receiving of comfort from one another.

Our aims are basic in the simplicity that is the greatness of hospice: to actively minimize suffering, to care rather than cure, and to set goals in terms of people rather than disease. Hospice without medical direction and input will fail. The spiritual nourishment is magnificent, but the financial rewards and the emotional tightrope that one treads daily are far from attractive to our junior colleagues, which makes recruitment difficult.

Thus, there remains a need for more involved physician participation in a hospice program. We function both as a visible day-to-day leader and participant in the administration of the program. We perform not as an isolated pocket of authority but as a team player, sharing, supporting, and nourishing one another. We cannot tolerate a cult of death and dying, for to do so would mean failure to our patients. We exist outside the conventional care system; therefore, we act as a liaison to other physicians who are not in synchrony with hospice philosophy. We act as educators and, one hopes, role models to our resident physicians, to medical students, to nurses and to social workers. We encourage and insist upon an open-door policy for learning, so that we may better recruit in the future and educate in the present. Dr. Sylvia Lack, who worked at both St. Joseph's Hospice and St. Christopher's Hospice in London, England, came to our shores and developed Hospice, Incorporated in New Haven, Connecticut in 1971 [4]. Dr. Lack identified ten commandments of hospice care, which are as follows [3]:

1. Coordinated home care with inpatient beds under a central autonomous hospice administration
2. Control of symptoms (physical, sociological, psychological, and spiritual)

3. Physician-directed services (due to the medical nature of symptoms)
4. Provision of care by an interdisciplinary team
5. Services available 24 hours a day, seven days a week, with emphasis on availability of medical and nursing skills
6. Patient and family regarded as the unit of care
7. Provision for bereavement follow-up
8. Use of volunteers as an integral part of the interdisciplinary team
9. Structured personnel support and communication systems
10. Patients accepted into the program on the basis of health care needs rather than their ability to pay

THE PATIENT IN PAIN—THE FAMILY IN PAIN

Our patients, families, and friends seek the lamp of sanctuary after a long and agonizing journey. Virgil, in his *Aeneid*, gives his hero a glimpse of those in the process of dying. Their transition has been interrupted and they plead for help (*tendebantque manus ripae ulteriorsis amore*): "They stretch out their hands with pleading and longing for the further shore."

So these patients appeal to us.

It would appear that the cyclical roller coaster of crisis, interventions, agonizing decisions, and a Niagara of frustrations is brought to hospice with a spark of hope. There is an ever-present fear and uncertainty as to what lies ahead. "Can I be further disfigured?" "Will I lose control?" "Dear God, give me a safe journey and release me from this torture and agony, this constant pain." "Doctor, can you help me die?" "Doctor, must we stand by and let him suffer?" "Doctor, can you put him out of his misery?" Pain, suffering and death are the unspoken companions that engulf the cancer patient and the family. Are these twentieth-century lepers to be regarded as a sign of failure, or is there a greater challenge for care when cure is no longer possible? The focus of our attention on the dying and their care was sharpened by Dame Cicely Saunders [4]. Her emphasis was to share, to communicate, and to facilitate being with one another. The control of pain was the glue that made all this possible. When the litany of euthanasia from friends, families, patients, and professional colleagues begins to assault your senses, keep questioning the quality of care we render.

The physician in hospice has to approach the patient in pain as a fireman responding to a four-alarm blaze. It is not important at this point to determine the origins of the fire, but it is important to contain it and extinguish it quickly.

Many of our patients come from homes where the burden of dying has been exhausting to the family or from a home without an accessible family or friend network. Many are transfers from other institutions, where the skills of hospice team cannot be brought to the patient's bedside. There is still within our society, especially prevalent among physicians and nurses, an orthodox arrogance that permits pain as a terminal event to exist—pain that is torture to the patient and scarring to the family and friends, pain that oftentimes does not permit death with dignity, pain that slows the healing and creates emotional scars in the survivors. We work on a priority scale,

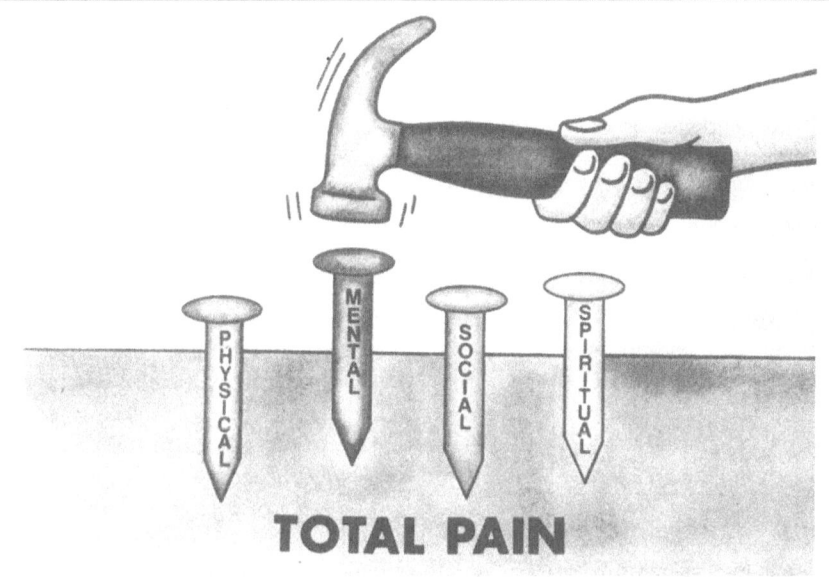

Figure 11-1. Pain to the cancer patient.

with the management of controlling pain assuming precedence over all other concerns. It is to this problem that we bring the full thrust of our caring team.

In his recent challenge to hospice programs, Dr. Balfour N. Mount stated,

A high order of clinical competence is essential if abuse of hospice is to be avoided.... Too often there is inadequate knowledge of pharmacology and pharmacokinetics, inadequate knowledge of neurology and medical oncology. In hospice, one thing we do not need is another way to do it badly. Medical incompetence by any other name is still medical incompetence [5]

The meaning of pain to the cancer patient is a total agony encompassing physical, emotional, spiritual, and financial components (figure 11-1). Hospice pain is an emergency, and all of our resources must be brought to the patient's bedside, since the patient is truly dying now and unfortunately will not come back later to die on our terms. Listen to the patient: it is his pain, not yours.

We treat each family as a unit, and must respond to its needs in a sensitive manner. The family unit acts as a guide communicating to us the fluctuating needs of the patient. Failure to respond to these sensitive signals at this time can wreak havoc with the treatment plan of this final phase of life.

Patient evaluation

Initially, and throughout the patient's stay, we do not hesitate to sit on the patient's bed, reach out and touch the patient, and then openly discuss the needs and priorities of care. We attempt to discuss death in a rational straightforward manner and then answer the family's burning questions. We do not answer questions as to remaining time for the patient.

A review of the previous medical records is made and a physical examination with care and gentleness is then carried out. We are especially concerned with early pressure sores or obvious decubiti: pruritus and subsequent excoriation; herpetic lesions; dehydration; oral candidiasis; dyspnea and cough; intestinal colic and obstruction; constipation; ascites; bladder spasm; bleeding sites; depression and anxiety; and increased intracranial pressure. Unfortunately, due to the prolonged stay in bed, patients present us with problems in myofascial pain and weakness.

It is important for us to determine the severity and the sites of pain. The patient or the family can assist in location of pain, which we mark on our anatomic drawing. The use of a 0–10 scale (0 being no pain, 10 being excruciating pain) is helpful to us in determining our progress in the relief of the patient's pain.

At the conclusion of the examination, we have to make some promises and then deliver immediately. Sleep, which has been obviously lacking, is readily accomplished with titratable liquid antidepressants. The relief of pain at rest, and then the relief of pain with movement are more difficult, but usually attainable with rational pharmacological tailoring of appropriate analgesics and other medications.

It is imperative at the conclusion of the examination to sit with the patient's primary care nurse and methodically go over the care plan. The ability of the hospice nurse at the bedside to act as an onsite extension of the physician always works to the best interest of the patient. We therefore provide, for the nurse's discretion, wide latitude and range of medications, with appropriate alternative routes of administration.

THE MANAGEMENT OF PAIN

The management of pain in the hospice patient is considerably different from that of the still-active cancer patient (figure 11-2). Over 60% of our admissions present with pain, and usually most have more than one pain. The cocoon of despair that envelops a poorly treated patient and family is readily apparent. In most instances there has been a multiplicity of failed treatment strategies: surgical, chemotherapy, and radiation. All too often polypharmacy has been tried and has compounded the problems facing the patient.

In hospice, because of the dying process, we are denied the luxury of time. Therefore, our resources must be brought to bear immediately. Unfortunately, due to the widespread underutilization of appropriate analgesics, unrelieved pain further erodes the patient's confidence in the medical system, thus bringing their dying into sharper focus. The withholding of analgesics for fear of addiction cannot be tolerated in hospice, and in most instances there is no ceiling placed on analgesic dosing.

As seen in figure 11-3, a ladder of pharmacological steps can be climbed to relieve the suffering. The greater majority of our patients have progressed over time from the peripheral-acting nonnarcotic analgesics to the major narcotic agonists, either the lesser potent agents (codeine, proproxyphene, or oxycodone) or the strong narcotic agonists (morphine, methadone, levorphanol, and hydromorphone). We do not use

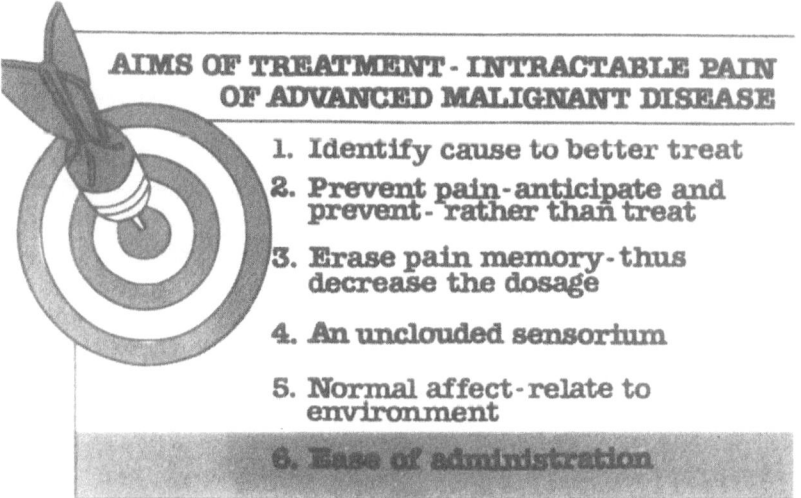

AIMS OF TREATMENT - INTRACTABLE PAIN OF ADVANCED MALIGNANT DISEASE

1. Identify cause to better treat
2. Prevent pain-anticipate and prevent-rather than treat
3. Erase pain memory-thus decrease the dosage
4. An unclouded sensorium
5. Normal affect-relate to environment
6. Ease of administration

Figure 11-2. Management of cancer pain in the hospice patient.

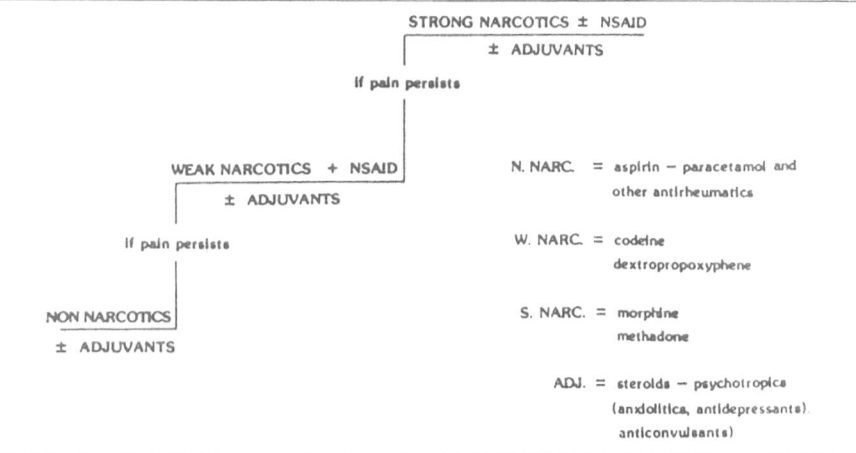

STRONG NARCOTICS ± NSAID
± ADJUVANTS

If pain persists

WEAK NARCOTICS + NSAID
± ADJUVANTS

If pain persists

NON NARCOTICS
± ADJUVANTS

N. NARC. = aspirin — paracetamol and other antirheumatics

W. NARC. = codeine
dextropropoxyphene

S. NARC. = morphine
methadone

ADJ. = steroids — psychotropics (anxiolitics, antidepressants), anticonvulsants)

Figure 11-3. Pharmacological steps to relieve cancer pain. Reprinted by permission of the World Health Organization.

the narcotic agonist—antagonist agents (pentazocaine, nalbuphine, butorphanol, buprenorphine), which have a very narrow therapeutic window as well as side effects that are usually unacceptable to the patient. In hospice, we prefer oral liquid morphine sulfate, since it has a wide margin of safety, spares the patient further discomfort of injections into wasted muscles, and, should the patient go home, provides him with a sense of independence in taking his own medications.

We find that oral liquid morphine sulfate, flavored to taste preference, served cold, and given by the clock every four hours, is most practical. The plasma half-life of morphine sulfate permits a practical four-hour schedule. Initially we give wide ranges of doses, from 5–60 mg or more if needed. The patient is awakened during the night until we reach a steady state; then we can double the sleep dose and permit an uninterrupted night's sleep.

Meperidine is the least acceptable choice in hospice pain management because of its short half-life and, more importantly, the unacceptable adverse effects of its metabolite, normeperidine, on the central nervous system. These effects include tremor, twitch, agitation, and convulsions. Patients with renal dysfunction will exhibit an increase in central nervous system effects when placed on meperidine.

Methadone, a potent opiod, is difficult to use, and unless the staff understands its unusual pharmacokinetics, the outcome can be disastrous for the patient. Because of a cumulative half-life of well over 50 hours, toxic plasma levels can occur even in the absence of adequate analgesia.

The average new admission can be controlled with a range of morphine sulfate from 5–40 mg on a routine four-hourly schedule, but with the understanding to the patient that we have no ceiling as to the amount of medication he can take. It is important to provide additional medication should pain occur prior to the next scheduled dose. One can safely use one half of the oral dose of morphine sulfate subcutaneously or provide additional oral dose of morphine sulfate between the scheduled four hours. We instruct our nurses to quickly escalate the starting dose by 50% if there are two or more breakthrough pains in 24 hours.

As an alternative route for morphine sulfate in patients who cannot swallow, the rectal route can be used. We use morphine sulfate, available in 5-, 10-, and 20-mg suppositories, hydromorphone 3-mg suppositories, or oxymorphone 5-mg suppositories. The dosage is the same as the oral route. Subcutaneously our preference is usually one third the oral route. Intravenously, we can start a continuous drip or give bolus injections. The drip is preferable, and it is usually one fourth to one third the oral dose. The epidural route is to be discussed later. The patient who cannot swallow either on admission or in the final phase of dying would certainly be a candidate for any of these parenteral routes. It would be cruel to abruptly stop the analgesic and precipitate even a mild form of withdrawal for the lack of using any of the alternative routes.

Intravenous morphine sulfate is used on rare occasions in hospice for the patients who are out of control with pain, cannot swallow, and have no rectum. In such cases, this becomes the technique of necessity. Our starting range is 0.5 mg to 10 mg/hr with escalation by 1-mg increments to achieve a level of comfort. It is suggested that the hourly intravenous dose be set at one fourth to one fifth that of the hourly oral dose.

Subcutaneous opiods are used either by intermittent injections or with a lightweight battery-operated pump [6]. We have elected to use hydromorphone, since it is more soluble than morphine sulfate in equianalgesic doses, thereby reducing volume. The specially developed 27-gauge insulin needle makes for patient comfort with this technique. There is an improvement in mobility for the patient, and the maintenance for the family is relatively simple compared to a continuous intravenous infusion. Insertion sites are the upper abdomen, between the scapulae and above the breasts. The needle is covered with a sterile adherent dressing (Opsite, Tegaderm) and changed either weekly or when needed.

No doubt we have not heard the last of the Congressional controversy over the use of diamorphine (heroin) in terminally ill patients. The Canadian government has recently approved the compassionate usage of heroin.

As a result of firsthand experience during two tours in English hospices, this author is convinced of the need for heroin in the dying. The drug is highly soluble, and a small volume of concentrated solution placed in a Graseby portable syringe driver provides comfort, a sense of euphoria, and ease of administration for the patient and the staff.

Guidelines to jog the brain

1. When changing to intravenous morphine infusion from oral usage, it is preferable to use one fourth to one fifth of the hourly oral dose. For example, if the patient was receiving 20 mg of oral morphine every four hours, the patient would then receive 5 mg per hour. Therefore, one fifth of the five would equal 1 mg, which would be a start for an intravenous infusion dose. We usually give a loading dose of IV morphine sulfate prior to the infusion; thus 1–2 mg or more IV push would be appropriate.
2. When changing from the oral route to the subcutaneous or intramuscular, we use one third to one half of the oral dosage. If the patient was receiving 20 mg every four hours, one half of 20 mg would be 10 mg sub q. or IM. The subcutaneous dose and the intramuscular dose are similar. The intravenous dose is slightly less than the intramuscular dose.

Epidural opiates

Epidural opiates are little used in hospice, but when feasible can provide a high degree of comfort. Unfortunately, patients and family at this stage of the dying process may be adamantly opposed to further invasive techniques. We have, however, inserted epidural catheters in home-care patients within the patient's home, and the families have been outstanding in their willingness to perform the needed daily injections.

Side effects of narcotics

Should there be somnolence or excessive tiredness, which is not uncommon early on with morphine sulfate, a reduction in the dose by 50% is indicated. The family and the patient should be forewarned of the possibility of an early sedative effect. When one considers the insomnia and fatigue with which most patients present, it is likely that the patient may be simply catching up on sleep deprivation. Should there be a persistence of somnolence, we add to the regimen at 0800 hours and 1200 hours 2.5 mg of liquid dextroamphetamine.

Nausea may be an early problem with start-up narcotics. Therefore, we add to every other dose of morphine sulfate in the first 48 hours 2.5 mg of liquid prochlorperazine.

It is a common mistake to discontinue the nonnarcotic analgesics with the step-up to the narcotic analgesics, but we continue to take advantage of peripheral-acting nonnarcotics such as acetaminophen, aspirin, and ibuprofen.

Constipation is an unfortunate companion to the opiods. This is the major complication of the use of opiod in hospice. It must be treated vigorously. Prior to the initiation of opiods, a rectal examination should be performed and appropriate measures instituted, which may include oral cathartics with stool softeners, enemas, suppositories, or manual removal of fecal impaction. The continuation of combined cathartics and stool softeners is important to the success of opiod use. Frequent inspection of the rectum should be made since impaction may exist with diarrhea. Some problems in opiod use are

1. Constipation
2. Nausea
3. Confusion and hallucinations
4. Dizziness
5. Initial drowsiness
6. Respiratory depression
7. Agitation or delirium

Confusion and hallucinations may be seen early. Especially in older patients, we prefer to use haloperidol in a range of 0.5 to 20 mg qd. Thus hallucination usually clears, but if it should persist, our choice would be to switch to another opiod, preferably hydromorphone. One of the benefits of haloperidol, of course, is that it is a very potent antiemetic.

The potential for respiratory arrest is everpresent with scheduled dosing of narcotics as illustrated in the following anecdote. An 80-year-old nun who had an extensive tumor had been on one 50-mg meperidine tablet daily at home. When admitted to hospice, she was started on oral morphine sulfate 10 mg q 4 hourly. In a short time she manifested obvious signs of opiod overdose: respirations were eight per minute, pin-point pupils and unarousable coma. The family, after discussion of the situation and given choices, elected to permit the use of naloxone—the opiod antagonist. A dilute solution of naloxone 0.4 mg diluted to 10 ml with normal saline was administered in small increments. The respiratory depression was lifted, the patient responded with adequate analgesia, and the family was happy for those last few days of quality time together.

The use of oral opioids is most effective in the hospice environment, and this may be the magic of hospice. There is constant attention to detail by a caring team of professionals. There is reassurance to the patient and family that pain can and will be controlled. This represents the non invasive procedures which permit us to control pain. A number of things can be done for the patient who is in hospice that do not

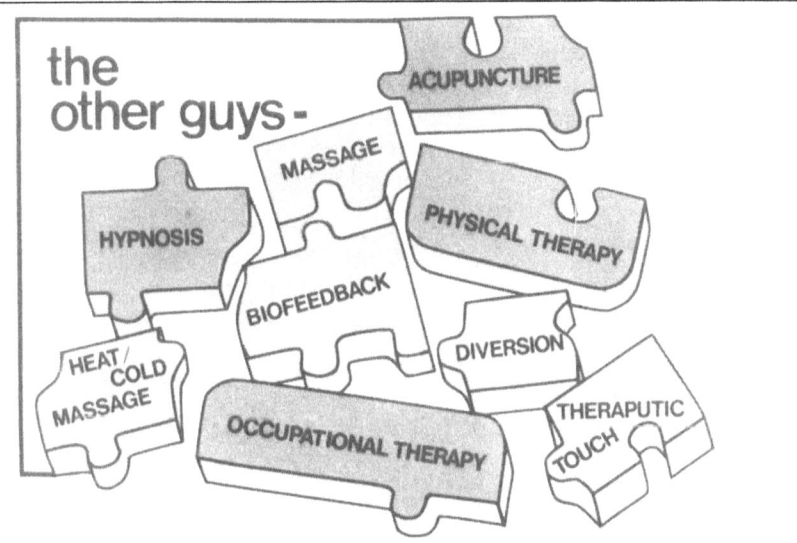

Figure 11-4. Nonpharmacological modalities to relieve cancer pain.

represent invasive procedures. Clinically speaking, the patients who are chronically medicated with narcotic analgesics often respond less favorably to nonpharmacologic modalities, which include acupuncture, hypnosis, transcutaneous electric nerve stimulation (TENS), therapeutic touch, biofeedback, imagery, relaxation, massage, vibration, spray, heat, and cold (figure 11-4). We can also include music therapy. Each one of these modalities represents a skill that the individual who comes to the bedside must understand and believe in. Thus may the patient have a successful journey. The basis of this entire noninvasive group is one of distraction with a very meaningful interaction between patient and therapist.

The procedures mentioned in figure 11-5 are, unfortunately, rarely called upon in hospice. They are used with discretion and understanding both with the patients' and families' permission. The ones that would be used most frequently would probably be the autonomic nerve blocks, the trigger-point injections, and the epidural opiods.

Progression of choice medications

Moving up the ladder from nonopiods to weak opiods to strong opiods, one must include adjuvant medication in order to be truly successful in the care of cancer patients. Under the adjuvant medications, one could list the following:

1. Anticonvulsants
2. Neuroleptics
3. Anxiolytics
4. Antidepressants
5. Corticosteroids

Type of Procedure	Most Common Indications
Nerve block	
Peripheral	Pain in discrete dermatomes in chest and abdomen
Epidural	Unilateral lumbar or sacral pain
	Midline perineal pain
	Bilateral lumbosacral pain
Intrathecal	Midline perineal pain
	Bilateral lumbosacral pain
Autonomic	
Stellate ganglion	Reflex sympathetic dystrophy (e.g., frozen shoulder)
	Arm pain
Lumbar sympathetic	Reflex sympathetic dystrophy
	Lumbosacral plexopathy
	Vascular insufficiency of the lower extremity
Celiac plexus	Midabdominal pain
Continuous epidural infusion with local anesthetics	Unilateral and bilateral lumbosacral pain
	Midline perineal pain
Chemical hypophysectomy	Diffuse bone pain
Inhalation therapy	Generalized pain
	Incident pain
Trigger-point injection	Focal muscle pain

Figure 11-5. Types of anesthetic procedures commonly used for cancer pain. Reprinted by permission of the New England Journal of Medicine. Foley, KM. The treatment of cancer Pain, 1985; 313: 84–95.

Our anticonvulsant of choice would either be phenytoin or valproic acid; our neuroleptic of choice would be haloperidol; our anxiolytics of choice would be diazepam and alprazolam; our antidepressant of choice would be doxepin, for the simple reason that it comes as a liquid concentrate and we can titrate better; our corticosteroid of choice would either be prednisone or dexamethasone. Our use of antiemetics has been appreciably enhanced with the use of haloperidol 0.5 mg PO t.i.d. or parenterally 5 mg t.i.d. We use prochlorperazine liquid, 2.5 mg with every other morphine dose for the first 48 hours, after which it is usually not needed.

For severe intractable vomiting we have had some success with the use of scopalamine ear patches which are good for 72 hours. This provides an antiemetic effect and in some patients a welcome sedative effect. Occasionally some patients respond to ginger capsules or drinking ginger ale as needed.

Many of our patients are elderly or debilitated and have difficulty in swallowing. Controlled studies of many of the adjuvant drugs with cancer patients are lacking.

One must not prescribe adjuvant drugs routinely; rather, the choice of the drug should always be dictated by the individual patient and his needs. In order to avoid the calamity of excessive sedation and possibly coma, one must use homeopathic dosages of these drugs. Even in small doses, the effect sometimes is welcome and profound. Chlorpromazine is a profound antiemetic, but it may be too potent a sedative. For sedation, we prefer, at times, to use rectal diazepam, which we have learned to make from English hospice. It is now being prepared in our hospital pharmacy in 10-mg strength. The use of haloperidol, as previously stated, represents our first line of choice both for its ability to clear up the confusional state from opioids and for its antiemetic effect. There may be an analgesic effect that perhaps is more visible in the terminally ill patient than in other patients. The drug seems to have a de facto analgesic effect on emotional upheaval. Haloperidol is also for us a less sedative drug with fewer anticholinergic and cardiovascular effects than chlorpromazine.

The use of anxiolytics, with alprazolam and diazepam being our first line of defense, are of great benefit, especially with acute anxiety and panic attacks. These are common problems especially in pulmonary metastatic disease or primary disease of the lung, where there is an intense feeling of suffocation. We have resorted to the use of diazepam suppositories or oral diazepam combined with intravenous morphine to lessen the problems of suffocation, which the patients describe very vividly to us.

The use of the corticosteroids in hospice are primarily for patients with headache from raised intracranial pressure and for patients with bone pain. Beneficial effects of corticosteroids include appetite stimulation and mood enhancement. The steroid medications also are useful in relieving pain associated with nerve compression and spinal cord compression. Both prednisone and dexamethasone are equally effective (note that 1 mg of dexamethasone is equivalent to 7 mg of prednisone). Nonsteroidal antiinflammatory drugs, with their antiprostaglandin effect, are especially useful for bone pain. Prior to the withdrawal of zomepirac (Zomax) by McNeil Pharmaceutical, this was our first drug of choice. At the present time, we are using ibuprofen.

We have recently observed in London hospice that the use of calcitonin in the treatment of bone pain had modest success in abating this excruciating symptom. The suggestion that salmon calcitonin is helpful in reducing bone pain has been described extensively. There is a suggestion of an increase in betaendorphin circulating levels seen only in patients treated with salmon calcitonin [1]. We are using 100 units subcutaneously once a day. Skin testing to rule out allergic reactions is simple to do, but should be mandatory.

Whenever prolonged, constant, or intermittent pain cannot be relieved by removing the cause or by administration of potent analgescis, it is termed *intractable*. This type of pain is a feature of cancer. When intractable pain causes an unacceptable degree of physical or mental stress uncontrolled by simple analgesics, a critical review of all aspects of the problem should be undertaken as follows:

1. Removal of the source of pain may be impossible because (a) it cannot be identified: or (b) the primary disorder is too extensive (for example, in multiple metastases); or (c) it would involve an unacceptable risk to the patient's life; or (d) it would result in severe disability or disfigurement.
2. While the use of some powerful analgesics may accelerate the patient's deterioration, careful selection of potent analgesics will relieve pain and preserve mental activity.
3. Since intractable pain is often a feature of terminal illness, proper management of the dying patient is of great importance. This demands sympathy and understanding and often the use of tranquilizers, coanalgesics, antidepressants and other drugs. It must be added here that no drug is an adequate substitute for human compassion.
4. In certain cases, drug treatment is inappropriate either because it is ineffective or because it impairs the patient's physical and mental well-being.

HOSPICE TEAM

The opportunity for patient and family to begin the grieving process is of great importance in our multidisciplinary approach. Each member of our group brings finely honed skills to the bedside. We are a hospital-based hospice with the advantage of a building separate from the main hospital. We have the best of two worlds, in that we have inpatient care for those who are truly out of control and cannot be managed at home. We also have a 24-hour-a-day, seven-days-a-week home-care service, with a phone that is always manned by knowledgeable nurses who have the needed skills to respond to the cancer patient and to the family in distress.

Bereavement is uppermost in our minds as the dying process continues. Our early warning radar alerts us to families who may need further support after the death of a loved one. Each team member is assigned a role in bereavement follow-up for at least six months. It has been said that grief is the price paid for love. A memorial service at St. Mary's Hospice Chapel is held every three months with the bereaved families, friends, and staff. We make efforts to avoid the anger, the isolation, the guilt, and the confusion that takes place. Drugs should be used sparingly to soften the grief except in the case of the true symptom complex of an unrelieved depression. Personal phone calls, visits, and letters are important in extending our work beyond death. We have seen drug problems, alcoholism, and death in a small percentage of the surviving family. The hospice team has an unwritten contractual relationship to provide support in the bereavement period. If there is discord in the dying phase, bereavement can be enhanced grief. The discord, of course, can be lack of attention to and the inadequate care of the myriad symptoms that seem to overwhelm both patient and family. There needs to be an effective and affectionate relationship between the team and the family unit.

We are open to the family and to the patient. We do not give time tables for dying; we do not prioritize our time to care for the sickest and neglect the less sick. We work on quality time. At times, the anger and frustration surface in volcanic emotional eruptions that literally exhaust and challenge our skills as fellow human beings. We provide the conduit and hopefully can continue to listen to the raging.

Do not go gentle into that good night,
Old age should burn and rave at close of day;
Rage, rage against the dying of the light.

(Dylan Thomas)

The weekly staff meeting is opened with a prayer for our patients who have died. We each take turns in reciting some uplifting words, be it biblical, poetic, or musical. This sets a tone of togetherness, and the harmony provides some of the thread that holds us as one. Discussions on a medical, social, and psychological level are held on problem patients and families. This open forum enables us to blend each of our skills to the benefit of the family unit.

The medical director of a hospice unfortunately walks a very fragile tightrope. It is fragile in the sense that there is a love–hate relationship with referring physicians: love, in that referring physicians are deeply appreciative of the support and expertise that we can offer the patient; and perhaps hate because we succeed very quickly where their knowledge has not permitted them to achieve immediate results in the management of the terminally ill.

As medical director, I am responsible for the quality of care delivered to all of the patients in our 10-bed unit. My operating-room background did not prepare me in the ways of hospice. The six c's, which should be standard in all medicine, are especially needed in hospice. They are competence, concern–compassion, comfort, communication, and cheerfulness.

As a Pain Management Specialist, I can bring needed skills to the bedside to better manage pain. I have made a quantum leap as an anesthesiologist from the technical world of the operating room to the bedside of the dying, where the challenges never end and the skills are under constant refinement.

Our nursing staff represents the epitome of acute palliative care skills. It is they who 24 hours daily bear the primary responsibility for patient care. If you will, they are the mirror image of the physician at the bedside.

The pastoral care member is a Catholic nun, who provides spiritual ecumenical care to all. For her, death is a reality and this attitude eases the burden of patient and family. To all, she is a source of strength and comfort.

The social worker stands tall in the many tasks we always seem to find for him. There is a neverending blizzard of paper work, be it financial, insurance, placement, transfer, or legal, but he seeks the best path for the family. We have expanded the conventional role of social work with counseling and bereavement follow-up. We have many problems with families and friends who lack support during this trying time. Our social worker puts his oar into the troubled waters and assists where needed.

Our dietician brings knowledge, imagination, and creativity to both our inpatient population and those on home care. The difficulty of even providing minimal calories in the face of starvation, dehydration, and protein calorie malnutrition taxes her imagination. Anorexia, oral candidiasis, and the terrible taste in this final stage are challenging and many times cannot be overcome.

Our physical and occupational therapists work in concert with us, not so much in the tradition of rehabilitation but rather by offering some hope in the management of tasks we take for granted. Rising from bed, shaving, or combing one's hair can be taxing and frustrating to the patient with atrophied muscles and metastatic disease. The therapists gently soothe and try to accomplish in a short period of time some function, endurance, and hopefully increased safety.

The secretary of the unit bends her skills to the wheel of our common goal. She conveys a sense of giving and cheerfulness to the first-time patient and visitor. It must be this way, since she is usually the first voice they contact.

Our volunteers, bless them, are the pure givers. Often they are taken for granted, but they are unsung heroes and heroines who share their precious time and energy with the dying patient. These dedicated civilians are screened and taught the ways of hospice. The commitment to listen, to help, and to return to the bedside of the dying is their major contribution.

There are difficulties with families who rage and with patients who, unfortunately, cannot accept the dying process. Staff breakdown may result from the erosion of emotions after long hours in dealing with this unique group of patients.

CONCLUSON

As Henry VanDyke has written, "Time is too slow for those who want, too swift for those who fear, too long for those who grieve, too short for those who rejoice, but for those who love, time is an eternity." Hospice is a loving affair in the final phase of life. As it is written in Jewish wisdom, "Better one deed than a thousand sighs."

ACKNOWLEDGMENT

Our hospice at St. Mary's Hospital in Milwaukee, Wisconsin is located in a landmark hospital building overlooking Lake Michigan. St. Mary's Hospital is an integral part of the Daughters of Charity. This order was founded in France in 1633 and established in the United States in 1809. The beacon of love and care which is acute intensive palliative care is a commitment of the Daughters. Sister Julie Hanser, our administrator, has been gracious in her support of the hospice and its philosophy.

There are special thanks to be rendered to the people who made my hospice journey possible: my dear wife, an extraordinary and loving companion in life's journey who shares with me the joy and sadness of hospice, and our family, who constantly remind me to look forward to each day for it is life; Sister Harriet Copperman at North London Hospice, London, England, a friend and teacher; Dr. Beverley Britt, Professor of Anesthesia at the University of Toronto, a dear friend who assisted in the birthing process of this manuscript at her home in Wales; my staff, and the patients and their families, without whom hospice at St. Mary's could not exist; my personal secretary, Renee Gerlach, always a welcome voice of comfort, care and support to all of our patients and to me, who blended her skills, unlimited time, and effort to enable my mission to flourish; my chiefs, Drs. John P. Kampine and Stephen E. Abram at the Medical College of Wisconsin, who afforded me the privilege of blending compassion and knowledge in a teaching environment; and Fr. John Sheehan, S.J. at Marquette University, dear friend, severe critic, guide, and teacher in the paths of preparation of this manuscript.

REFERENCES

1. Stenn F (1980): Thoughts of a dying physician. Forum on Medicine 3:718–719.
2. Aikenhead M (1914): The Letters of Mary Aikenhead. Dublin: M.H. Gill and Son Ltd.
3. Lack SA (1979): Hospice—A concept of care in the final stage of life. Connecticut Medicine 43:367–372.
4. Saunders CM (1978): The Management of Terminal Disease. Chicago: Year Book.
5. Mount B (1985): Challenges in palliative care. Keynote address. The American Journal of Hospice care 22–29.
6. Campbell CF, Mason JB, Weiler JM (1983): Continuous subcutaneous infusion of morphine for the pain of terminal malignancy. Ann Intern Med 98:51–52.
7. Gennari C, Agnusdei D, Civitelli R, Montagnani H (1984): Peripherally administered calcitonin and analgesia. XVIII Eur Symp Calc Tiss Angiers, ABS. No. 276.

INDEX